Praise for FROM **PUNK** TO **MONK**

"Ragunath's transformation shows how one person's choice to evolve can change the lives of so many. This book is real, funny, and inspirational."

—JAY SHETTY

"Ray's extraordinary journey is not only a testament to the power of principled living, but also a stirring call to be better stewards to the people around us. From Punk to Monk proves that keeping your heart and mind open can radically transform your life."

—RICH ROLL

"Raghunath is a beloved, enlightened teacher to countless people all over the world. The compassion and expertise in which he presents his music, yoga, and podcasts— along with his personal interactions—transforms our hearts and uplifts our spirits. I am sincerely grateful that in this book he is sharing his own extraordinary life. His story is filled with adventure, wisdom, and hope. Thank you, Raghunath."

—RADHANATH SWAMI

"Sincerity of heart is the golden road of Devotion. Like a flame dispelling darkness, Raghunath's heart has led him forward on the Path and shines out to help others find their way. Ram Ram."

—KRISHNA DAS

"I read this book in two days; I could not put it down. This is a story so relatable and compelling, filled with profound spiritual teachings presented not as dogmatic, lofty preaching, but as practical wisdom to help us navigate our day. Raghunath humbly shares his insights about how he learned that leading an authentic spiritual life has very little to do with following rules and adhering to do-nots; it is about the joy that arises from remembering God and being kind to others."

—SHARON GANNON, founder of Jivamukti Yoga

"From Punk to Monk *describes Raghunath's gritty journey of self-realization; a fascinating story of an American youth finding his home in Eastern tradition, through the rocky road of existential crises, ear-splitting music, and risk-filled adventures."*

—KELI LALITA, founder of Mantralogy Records and guitarist for 108

"From Punk to Monk *is an excellent contribution to the ever-growing body of literature on Krishna devotion in the West. Much of this literature prioritizes technical philosophical exposition, so it is a welcome relief to see Cappo's grass roots, nitty-gritty account of his own metamorphosis from a charismatic figurehead of the straight-edge movement to an equally charismatic teacher of yoga with major bhakti overtones. And this philosophy pervades the book in Cappo's inimitable, New York manner of straightforward but deeply wise exposition. Cappo has inspired many young seekers to explore and take up the path of bhakti, and, indeed, the value of spiritual autobiographies is nothing other than this: to provide a personal odyssey template that others can emulate in real life. This, Cappo has done, in an entertaining but deeply devotional way. A great read of a fascinating devotional journey, with an abundance of spiritual adventures all along the way."*

**—EDWIN BRYANT, Professor of Hindu Religion and
Philosophy, Rutgers University**

"As a fan, it's so interesting for me to learn about Raghunath's early years and how the punk community played a role in the search for the spiritual meaning behind playing music for people. I look up to him as a father and a singer, and I would recommend this book for anyone who is interested in hardcore music, spirituality, and self-discovery. Also, as an addict in recovery, reading about the ethics of the straight-edge community and the ideals behind it has helped me immensely in my journey."

—ANTHONY GREEN, lead singer of Circa Survive, Saosin, and L.S. Dunes

"I've known Ray Cappo since 1986, and I thought I knew him pretty well—until I read his book! The stories and adventures from his spiritual odyssey had my full attention. If you have any interest in tales about living on the outskirts of society, founding an outsider music scene, and allowing God to direct the course of your life, this book is for you."

—ANTHONY "CIV" CIVARELLI, lead singer of Gorilla Biscuits

FROM PUNK TO MONK

A MEMOIR

FROM PUNK TO

MONK

A MEMOIR

RAY RAGHUNATH CAPPO

FROM THE BANDS YOUTH OF TODAY AND SHELTER

FOREWORD BY MOBY

MANDALA

SAN RAFAEL LOS ANGELES LONDON

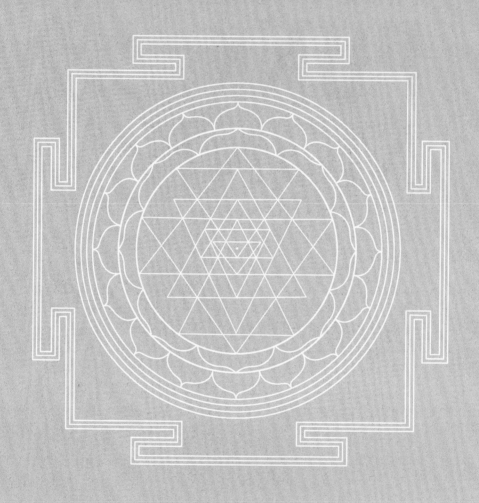

In the process of writing this memoir, I've realized that I have never been unattended or neglected. God has always sent teachers, mentors, friends, lovers, and children as guides to change the trajectory of my life. I remain in debt and grateful to all of you.

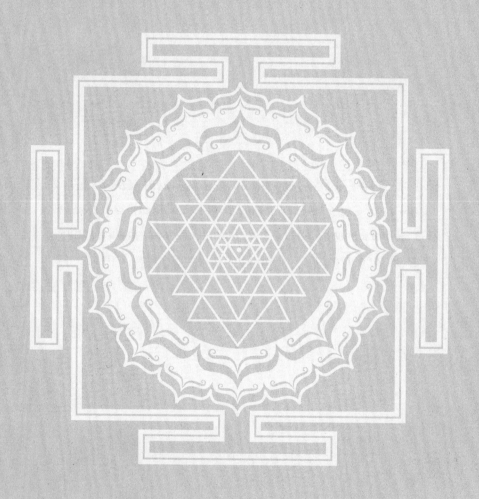

CONTENTS

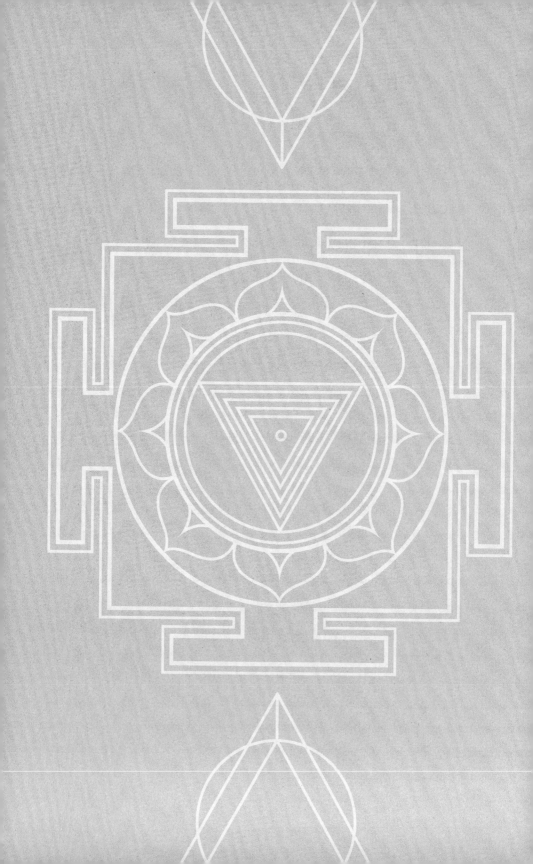

FOREWORD

It was the spring of 1983, and we were going to make $10 each playing a show, which was $10 more than any of us had ever made playing a show.

I was in the hardcore punk band Vatican Commandos, and Ray was in Reflex From Pain and Violent Children. Somehow, a student at Choate Rosemary Hall (a prep school with alumni like John F. Kennedy, Ivanka Trump, and Glenn Close, to name a few) had convinced the school to let him organize a spring concert. There was one catch. In order to get approval from the dean, we had to change our band names. So, Reflex From Pain became Reflections From Poetry, Vatican Commandos became Velvet Choices, and Violent Children became Violet Children. But even though our names had changed for the day, our music was still the loudest, fastest hardcore we could play.

We were *suburban* hardcore kids. By day, we attended high school in Connecticut. By night, we either watched TV with our parents or went to hardcore shows in Lower Manhattan, at the Anthrax in Stamford, or at Pogo's in Bridgeport. These cities hadn't been gentrified yet, and even downtown Stamford was a war zone.

We tried our best to be cool, to be tough, but when we went to A7 or the Great Gildersleeves or CB's in Lower Manhattan, we realized pretty quickly that we were little nerds who knew more about twentieth-century literature and how to sneak into country clubs than how to break into a squat on Avenue C.

Early '80s hardcore was our apprenticeship to music, to activism, to idealism. Hardcore was about celebration and community, but it was also about principles and ideas. You couldn't listen to Bad Brains and Minor Threat and Black Flag and Void and Dead Kennedys and not recognize that the status quos (fashion, politics, art, music, media, food, etc.) were all shallow and worthy of contempt. And hardcore was a true alternative. Sure, at times it was scary (Cro-Mags and Murphy's Law at Rock Hotel come to mind), but it was also thoughtful and principled. When you fell during a show, a bunch of hands reached down to pick you up. If you wanted to find out about ideas that were rationally radical, you just read lyric sheets or pamphlets at the merch table. And the best thing about hardcore? It was ours.

Music in the early '80s was corporate. Across the board. It was the Eagles and Michael Jackson and Steely Dan and Huey Lewis. Not bad, per se, but created by corporations to benefit corporations. Hardcore was truly DIY. Ray and Porcell and Vatican Commandos and all of the other hardcore kids in pretty much every suburb on the planet had to figure out how to do everything in order to play music and release records. We had to learn how to book shows, print flyers, make T-shirts, press vinyl, bring records to college radio stations, and so on. There was no infrastructure. We had to do it ourselves, or it wouldn't be done.

A few years after Ray and I became Violet Children and Velvet Choices at the Kennedy/Trump alma mater, I saw him at Angelica Kitchen in NYC. We'd both become vegetarians (and later, vegans), which made perfect sense to me. In the early '80s, when you started questioning the status quo, you invariably started questioning food. A quick look at the meat and dairy industries—and the world of Burger King and bacon and heart disease and suffering—will lead anyone with a rational/critical mind to realize that the culture around food production and consumption is horrifying.

As Ray rose to iconic status with Youth of Today and Shelter, I found myself both celebrating his success and being impressed that the underlying principles that had been instilled in us at hardcore shows in the early '80s hadn't waned. In fact, it seemed as if success had made Ray even *more* principled, which doesn't happen very often in life. Especially in the world of music.

Fast forward to 2019. I rented a car and drove to Upstate New York to interview Ray (and later in the day Porcell and Rob Zombie) for my *Punk Rock Vegan Movie*. We sat outside at his yoga farm, two guys in our early fifties who had both been on baffling and surprising and unprecedented musical and existential journeys. But underneath it all—not even buried very deep, it seemed—we were still sixteen-year-olds in Connecticut standing on the side of the stage at Pogo's, working up the nerve to stage dive while Bad Brains played "Banned in D.C."

MOBY

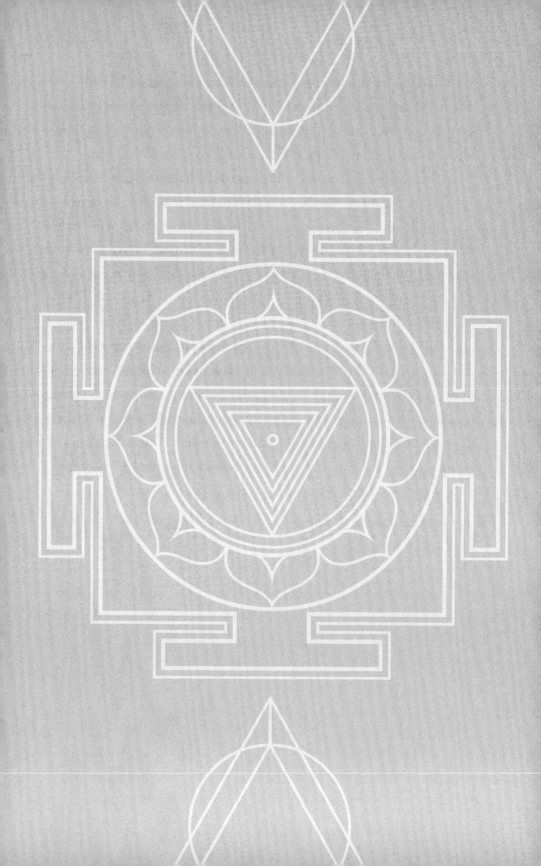

AUTHOR'S NOTE

Thank you for joining me on this pilgrim's journey. There are many more stories, travels, and people that transformed my life than appear in the pages of this book. I wanted to include them all, but my editors (understandably) trimmed things down. I've also intentionally changed some names. I apologize if you were a part of my journey and you aren't mentioned here. You are not forgotten.

In addition, the timeline may be out of sequence in places. I've tried my best to remember things in the order they happened, but my memory isn't perfect.

I especially want to thank all my friends and the fans of my music who've taken the messages of clean living, positivity, animal rights, and spirituality (none of which I claim ownership of) and have applied them to their lives. It's truly inspiring.

This lifetime is a blip. A moment in time. The blink of an eye. We are spirits made to love. Our choices either upgrade or degrade our consciousness, helping us evolve or moving us in a figure eight—learning the same lesson over and over until we graduate. I'm hoping this book will help you evolve.

I'm in debt to all the teachers, gurus, loved ones, and friends in my life, and of course, my growth accelerators—my children.

Remaining at your service,

RAY RAGHUNATH CAPPO

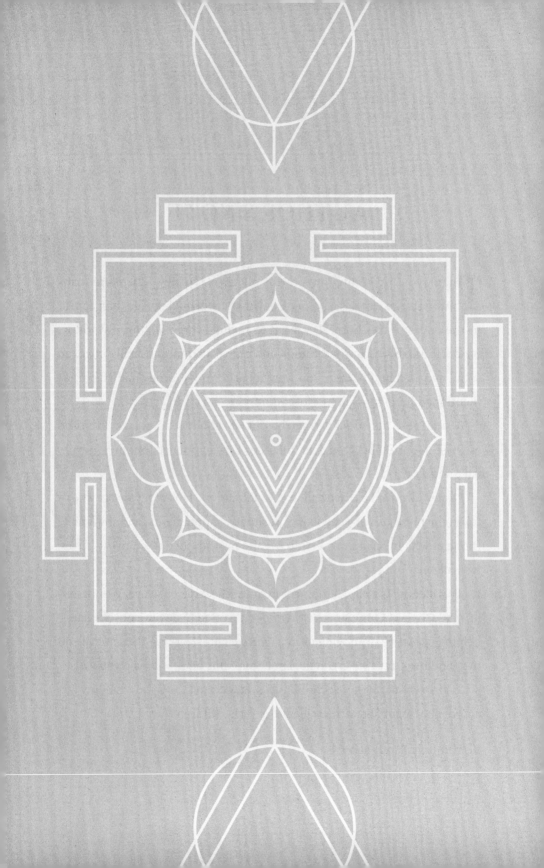

PROLOGUE

It was 2:30 a.m. in an empty warehouse parking lot in Buffalo, New York, and all I could feel or hear or see were the fists pummeling my face—punch after punch after punch—the silhouette of a gun pointed at me, a loud crack as something hard smashed into my head, then my knee, the taste of copper in my mouth, hot blood in my eyes. My legs gave way. I was vastly outnumbered and alone—my bandmates had fled, our stellar performance from earlier in the night long forgotten. I knew that I might not get out of there alive, and if I *did* survive, my body would be mangled and broken.

In that moment of helplessness, I did the only thing I knew how to do: I chanted the holy names of God, the Divine, the Absolute: "Krishna! Govinda! Rama! Madhava!" It seemed counterintuitive. Why not run? Why not fight? Instead, I sang. As if these mantras were being channeled through my body. My cries weren't as loud as the fists and the screams around me, but suddenly I felt completely safe, the *big* kind of safe. All my practice and seeking had prepared me for this.

I had been training for this moment for years.

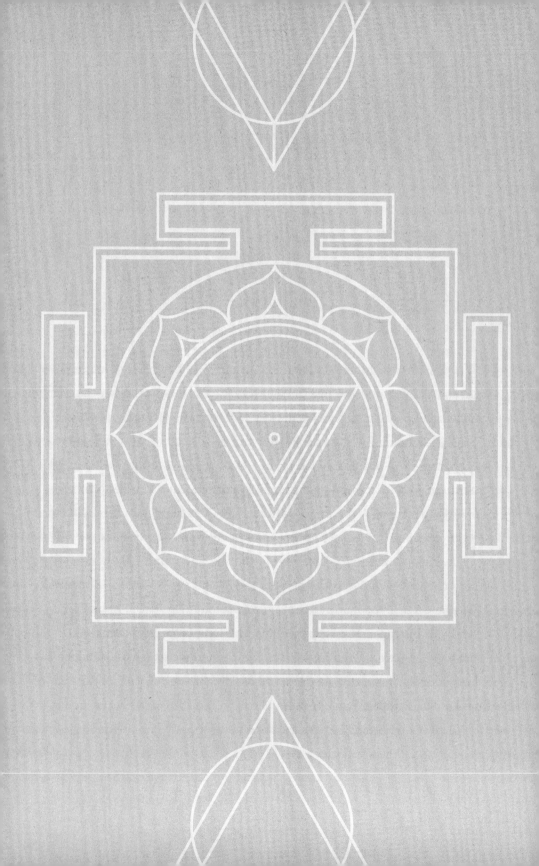

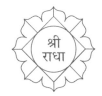

CHAPTER 1

INDIA, 1988

Ch-ch-ch-ch-ch-ch-ch-ch. As I sat in the third-class train to Kolkata, the steady, repetitive sound of iron wheels meeting the track of the Indian railway reminded me of a train from the 1930s, right out of an episode of *The Little Rascals*, which I'd watched as a kid. The train was probably as old as those episodes. It needed a good power washing and some bleach, but it was still exponentially more intriguing than the Metro-North train I used to take from Westchester to New York City. This was a punk-rock train. A total mess. Like India in 1988. Functioning chaos. And yet at the same time, this country had seemingly millions of social, religious, and superstitious rules that I didn't understand as an outsider. From my perspective, India was a hot-mess express with deep spiritual values. It was a lot like me.

I got to India in September 1988, when I was twenty-two years old. My father had just died after being in a coma for three years. Since I was fourteen, I'd been hanging out in New York City's Lower East Side and playing gigs on weekends, and I'd been touring with hardcore punk bands since I was sixteen. The disorder of the Lower East Side in the early 1980s prepared me to feel right at home in India. I was a teenage straight-edge, hardcore, yogic vegetarian on a quest for truth, God, and otherworldly love. Love with a capital *L*. Internal forces were pushing me to leave my world behind. I'd walked away from my family, my friends, my bandmates, my fans, and my entire music scene. I'd given my share of the record company I'd started to my high school friend and partner. I'd told him I had no interest in the music business. After signing twenty bands, I went from touring the United States with my hardcore band Youth of Today to being an all-in orthodox Hindu monk—well, almost all in. My excitement and determination vacillated daily, especially in those early days. I'd lost faith in the material world, yet there was so much to digest about how the culture of ancient India met modern-day Indian society. The philosophy and lifestyle were so foreign to me.

I didn't lament giving up my previous life as a frontman. In return, I'd received the greatest gift I could give myself: a rebirth. A clean canvas. A chance not to reinvent myself but to uncover what was already inside of me. I didn't go to India to put on a Hindu costume; I got into Vedic teachings to uncover all the costumes I'd been wearing and to find out what I was at my core. The sacred literature of India explained this in a way that gave me the broadest understanding of spirituality I'd ever had. I was ready to dive into the ocean of devotion, living in India with all its colors, scents, and raw beauty. I went straight to Krishna's holy land—Vrindavan—where Krishna, the young cowherd boy, the origin of all thirty-three million demigods, the Supreme Personality, had resided five thousand years ago in His manifestation on earth. The place was still alive. Vibrant. Totally inspiring.

But then, only a few months later, I left Vrindavan feeling like a loser because I couldn't make the cut. The power of that holy place and its holy people created a detoxifying effect. A purging. But I found the transformation too confrontational. I faced off against too many inner demons too quickly. I became critical, rude, intolerant, arrogant, and defensive. I lost perspective. Senior monks encouraged me to leave Vrindavan and go to an ashram in Kolkata, and perhaps visit the holy place of Mayapur a few hours north of the city.

So there I was on that third-class train, feeling crestfallen. After shaking off my bad attitude about this unexpected change of location, I decided to do something radical. I shifted my perspective. I exclaimed, "My life is in God's hands." I moved forward on my physical and spiritual journey, which was both an internal and external adventure.

The train trip from Delhi to Kolkata was twenty-five hours. There was no air conditioning, and it was hot. I tried to keep things in perspective. This was the cheap train, costing me about eight bucks. I was accompanied by five young Indians—four monks and one shop owner, Mohan, the brother of two of the monks. Mohan was shorter than me, dressed in a collared shirt and maroon sweater vest. He had a little mustache and short, black, sweaty hair combed over to the side. He wasn't a monk, but he believed it all. I, on the other hand, was new to this. Still hesitant. Questioning too much.

Mohan didn't look rich. But nobody in India did, even the rich. So I suppose he could have been. The monks barely spoke to me—not in a rude way; they were just focused on reading or chanting on their japa mala, which are like an Indian rosary. Although I understood, this appeared a little robotic and boring. I struggled with chanting japa, a meditative repetition of a mantra or divine name that is practiced in many Eastern spiritual traditions. Perhaps my mind was too busy. Perhaps that was a reason to take it more seriously.

If the monks were a little aloof, Mohan was the opposite. Overly engaging. Dramatic. He would get close to me and whisper, then speak loudly, waving his arms. He was touchy, too. Hugging for a few more seconds than I was expecting. And though he was generally positive and upbeat, he could turn pouty and somber at a moment's notice. But he was usually smiling. Big smiles, as if he were possessed by a happy clown. He stared deep into my eyes, asking me how I was feeling and what I was thinking.

The four young monks had all been in Vrindavan, at the same ashram where I'd been in residence. One of the brothers, Gopal, was the complete opposite of Mohan. He was introverted. He had little emotion and remained private. But he was a great cook, and right there, in the middle of the train, he uncovered a basket of kachoris, a delicious spicy puffed pastry filled with moong dal. He pulled out a stainless-steel pot.

"What's that?" I asked.

Mohan lit up. "Tamarind chutney!" He stamped his feet up and down like a happy child. I was excited, too. I hadn't brought anything to eat except for some Parle-G biscuits, a lightly sweetened sugar cookie that was a standard in Indian households and my go-to comfort food. The kachoris looked and smelled heavenly. My mouth watered just looking at them.

"Made with love and offered to Lord Krishna," Mohan said, smiling sweetly.

Indian people loved to snack, and their snacks were always homemade. Mohan reached into a bag and handed me a patravali, an ingenious biodegradable plate made from sal, or banyan leaves, delicately pinned together with toothpicks and cut into circles. Then he handed me a cup, similarly constructed. He carefully filled the cup with chutney and gave me three kachoris, which were still warm. Without saying any prayers, I dove in. After I devoured all three, Gopal put three more on my plate without even asking if I wanted them. (I did!) I enjoyed the Vedic style of eating with your hands. Actually, *hand*. The right hand was for clean things, and the left hand was for dirty things.

Now I was geared up for this train ride. Fed and ready for an adventure.

I was seated in the middle of the bench with one monk on either side and two more (plus Mohan) across from me. It was tight, but I felt I could do this. Twenty-five hours. Big deal. I would sleep for eight. Read a little. Chant a little. Eat some more kachoris. The squeaking of the train continued. I must have had two cups of that spicy tamarind chutney and ten or eleven kachoris. I don't do so well with "all you can eat."

I noticed that some people were getting on the train and not sitting. They were just standing there. Some were even sitting on the floor near the exit doors.

"Why aren't they sitting down in a berth like us?" I asked.

"They are very poor," Gopal said. "They have no money to sit."

I was appalled. "So they're going to sit on the floor of this dirty train for twenty-four hours?"

"You are right!" he said firmly. "It is very rude of us to not invite them to sit with us."

"No . . ." I said, backpedaling. "I wasn't saying—"

But Gopal was already motioning to them and telling them loudly to join us in our berth. I couldn't understand the Hindi, but it was some type of official invitation.

I tried to reason with him. "We're already packed in here. We can't fit any more."

But it was too late.

What had I done? Gopal was now helping them get comfortable in the berth. I said nothing, not wanting to seem whiny. Two old ladies were encouraged to sit on either side of me, sandwiching me even more tightly. The bench that was designed for three was now holding five. *This might go on for the next twenty-four hours!* I thought. Two more new people—older men, one with a massive turban that was taking up even more space—sat across from me. Mohan was in between them, facing me, as squished as I was. The kachoris in my stomach were officially churning. Something about the oil they were fried in wasn't sitting well. I was cramped and hot. I wasn't a happy camper.

Every culture has different ideas of personal space. In the United States, we tend to like a bit of room. But the ladies on either side of me didn't understand my needs. They were snuggling up to me, resting their heads on my shoulders.

The monk who'd invited them to sit with us felt good about the noble act of offering the poor a bit of bench at our expense. I, on the other hand, wanted to kick his ass for not asking me if I minded having two extra bodies beside me for the next twenty-four hours. I could feel the heat of the old ladies' bodies in the already ovenlike train. I was cracking.

Just then, an ancient lady—she looked to be two hundred years old and no more than five feet tall—walked onto the train, caught my eye, and eagerly walked toward me. She had an *om* symbol tattooed on her hand, coke-bottle glasses, and not a single tooth in her mouth. She squinted and pointed at me as if we knew each other. She was wrapped in a sari and carried a cheap duffle bag and a walking stick.

Where does she think she's going? I thought.

I couldn't look away. Our eyes were locked. She started yelling something in a language I didn't understand. I couldn't tell if she was cursing me or saying something sweet. But the people around us knew what she wanted. As she approached, I sat there transfixed, not knowing if she was happy, angry, or in excruciating pain. She got in my face, barked what sounded like an order, and stepped between my legs, hoisting herself up onto the luggage rack above my head.

All the monks were happy. They started chanting "Hari Bol," an Indian version of "Hallelujah."

I was shocked, but I figured so long as she remained out of my sight, I'd be okay, even though the other four people on my bench were pressing more firmly into me. As the old lady on the luggage rack got settled into a resting position, her skeletonlike arm draped over the side, dangling a few inches from my face.

I was losing it.

Two hours passed as I did my best to focus on the monks across from me, ignoring the women suctioned onto my shoulders. Sweat dripped from my brow, burning my eyes. The old ladies were also sweating. The heat was unbearable. Thick like a blanket. It had shut down my digestion. The kachoris just sat there in my stomach, fermenting. I didn't want to use the gross train bathroom. The toilet was an open hole to the tracks. *If there's a God in the sky, please help me,* I thought. *How many more hours of this? How can it get any worse?*

It could. And it did.

The train broke down in a field for what would end up being an eleven-hour delay. No air conditioning. No air to breathe. Packed with humans I didn't know. I was feeling queasy, and I was pretty sure I had a low-grade fever. The most fascinating thing was that nobody seemed to care—not the conductors nor the other passengers. Not the monks and not the travelers in my berth. Not the old lady sleeping in the luggage rack above my head. Nobody seemed to care except me. I cared a *lot*. I lost it. I went into blaming mode. I—a young, angry white monk—stormed around the train, searching for the conductor, or anyone in charge, and demanding accountability for the faulty system. Frustrated that nobody else was as upset as I was, I found myself saying out loud, like a mad man, "Doesn't *anybody* have anywhere to go except me?"

When I finally realized my efforts were futile and that everyone else was accepting what they couldn't control, I went back to my bench, squeezed into my seat, and sat down. I was defeated, but I wasn't quite ready to learn the lesson that was right in front of me.

Just like me, Mohan was flanked on both sides by strangers. Cramped. Hot. And for some reason, he was still wearing his sweater vest. *I'm sure he's uncomfortable*, I thought. Yet I seethed with envy. *Why can't I just be tolerant like him and all these other people? Why am I so damn entitled?* Mohan had every reason to complain, but he wasn't complaining. He was at ease. Everyone in this country seemed so much more tolerant and at peace than me.

This realization fueled self-loathing, which I promptly started projecting onto everyone else. Mohan was still bubbling with enthusiasm. Talkative. Spiritually enlivened. Bright-eyed. *Smiling.* But I found myself thinking that he was *too* enthusiastic, and I was growing increasingly annoyed. I wanted to complain and have others commiserate with me. That was my go-to attitude in tough times. But none of these people would commiserate. None of them had anything to complain about.

Mohan noticed my distress. He lifted his eyebrows. "Ra-aa-ay," he said in his singsong voice, making my name into a three-syllable word. This annoyed me even more. "What's the matter, Ra-aa-ay? You have been living in the holy town for some time now. You have so much knowledge, so much wisdom! You know that the material world is temporary and filled with pain. You know that we should be compassionate to all these souls." He pointed to my chest, voice dropping to a whisper. "You know the importance of compassion. To the degree we identify the body as the self, we will suffer." Then he fell silent, nodding his head theatrically. A real performer.

Unfortunately, he was giving advice to a person who couldn't hear it. I wanted to be angry and frustrated. I didn't respond.

"Ra-aa-ay!" Mohan said, smiling. "You have knowledge about the material realm, and you have some insight into the spiritual realm." He raised his voice so that people outside our berth could hear it. "You have a valuable gem! Live it! Give it! Look around this train, Ray!" He dropped to a whisper again. "The people are lost. Snacking. Gabbing. Sleeping. Talking nonsense. *You* have the power to inspire them. Change their hearts with transcendental sound."

I furrowed my brow. *What?*

He leaned closer. "We are alive for only a few years. A few decades if we're lucky. People are suffering in this world of samsara"—the cycle of birth and death and rebirth—"making the same mistakes again and again, but *you* have wisdom now, Ray. You must give it. You must give this wisdom away!" His smile and gaze were increasingly intense. I thought he might burst out laughing.

"What are you talking about?" I was dumbfounded. Disturbed. Sweaty.

"We must take the sacred sound of the Hare Krishna mantra," he bellowed, pointing his finger into the air, "and give it away freely to the entire train!"

"What?" I wanted him to keep his voice down.

"We must make the entire train chant the *Mahamantra*!" He stood up, beaming.

I still had no idea what he was talking about, but I wasn't in the mood for any of it. I glared at him, incredulous. "Do whatever you like, Mohan. Just leave me out of it."

He accepted this and went on his mission without me. He jumped onto one of the benches, holding on to the chains that supported the luggage racks. He leaned forward into the aisle. The train was lifeless, sitting there in the field, the usual mechanical clatter of the wheels absent. It was almost quiet.

"Our life is short!" Mohan addressed the packed train, speaking deeply, firmly, with hope in his voice. "There is so much time wasted! Let's not waste another moment! Let's all take this moment to glorify the divine Lord Krishna. He is the life of our life and the joy of our heart! His name is sweet like honey and is the medicine for the sleeping soul. Let's all invite Krishna's sweet, sacred name onto our tongues and into our minds and hearts! Let us sing and chant!"

Mohan reached into his pocket, pulled out karatalas—small cymbals—and skipped down the aisle, playing them and chanting the Hare Krishna mantra. He looked like a child joyfully bounding through a field.

I was shocked. Not because he was dancing freely and joyously, indifferent to public opinion. No, I was shocked because people started singing along. This would never have happened on New Jersey Transit. If someone said, "Let's get up and chant the holy name of Lord Krishna," people wouldn't even look up from their *New York Times*. But this was different. *Everybody* started singing, an impromptu chorus.

By the time the old women who were pressed into me started singing, I was no longer annoyed. I was happy. Even the old boney hand hanging in front of my face started clapping, rising in the air to meet another boney hand, hidden from view. Mohan continued dancing and singing like an actor in a musical leading a chorus. The most fascinating thing of all, though, was that *I* started singing. *I* started clapping. The power of the sound and the energy coming out of little Mohan lit me up. The mantra lit me up. That sacred sound vibration designed to call divinity into our lives lit me up. This unpretentious, five-foot-tall man, with his heart focused on God, lit up that entire train. Families were singing, the elderly were chanting, people were smiling and even dancing. He turned what could—*or even should*—have been a miserable experience into something I'll never forget. That chanting lasted at least an hour. People were swept up by this mantra that they all knew.

The *Mahamantra* is considered to be the most powerful of all mantras because it gives people what they need, not necessarily what they want. It's a mantra for trusting that our lives are in divine hands. A mantra that represents connection, and that reveals that we're part of a greater, divine plan. On that train trip, it was delivered with humility, enthusiasm, and joy at the perfect moment. It jolted everyone on that train out of their minds, their thoughts, their gossip, and the minutiae of their existence. It shook me, slapped me, and embraced me. It got me out of my complaining. My pity festival. My self-hatred and my bitterness.

I learned a great lesson that day. The sounds that are in your mind and flow out of your mouth will make you joyous or miserable. I was letting the negative sounds of my mind own me. Mohan changed all that with a mantra. I learned not just tolerance or acceptance for what I couldn't control; I learned that this mantra, delivered with the right attitude, brought joy. This is what previous masters had claimed, and this is exactly what happened. *One person with a good attitude can change many.* I was changed that day. I still am.

"The majority of my problems," I wrote in my journal that day, "don't come from anything external. Not the weather, not the government, not mistreatment, and not lack of resources. The majority of my problems are coming from my bad attitude. I need to be careful what I consume through my ears. After all, the sounds I put in become the sounds in my mind, which become the sounds flowing out of my mouth. All these sounds are creating me, for better or for worse."

* * *

Eleven hours after the train broke down, I heard and felt it come to life again. I was elated. At the next stop, the three women, including the one in the luggage rack, left my berth. This gave my body and mind some relief from the heat and the cramped conditions. At the following stop, though, my legroom disappeared again. A young man sat across from me, throwing his suitcase over my head onto the luggage rack. He was Indian, dressed cleanly but tacky by American standards, wearing a collared polyester shirt and jeans, unlike most people on the train, who wore traditional Indian clothing. He stared at me loudly, if there is such a thing. He looked confused. I was wrapped in a dhoti, a traditional robe that men in India wear. I hadn't shaved in weeks. I was wearing flip-flops, I had cracked feet, and I was holding on to a japa mala while chanting quietly to myself. I looked like a holy dirtbag. This man must have seen people like me on the streets of India many times, but perhaps not as young or as white. He was about my age, and he looked me in the eye, really close now that we were sitting knee to knee.

"White sadhu? Why, man? Why?" His tone was mocking rather than merely curious.

Sadhus are dedicated to a life pursuing God, and he was shocked that anyone would want to adopt the Vedic way of his ancestors, including renunciation, robes, and mantra meditation. I guessed by the way he was dressed that he idolized the West. I switched out of holy mode, ready to revert to my New York attitude and get in his face. But instead of acting out, I passed my test. The old me would have become loud and brash, if not violent, when people stepped up to me. I continued quietly chanting on my mala without answering. I remembered high school when people would say provocative and cruel things to me for being a punk and dressing weird. But still, I bit my tongue and mentally cut him up instead of saying what I thought.

Will I ever escape fools? I'm nine thousand miles away from home, I'm trying to be my best self, and God sends a fool to sit right in front of me. This guy is obviously charmed by Western culture. He's clueless that the American dream is a trap.

I breathed deeply to calm myself as he continued to stare at me.

Doesn't he understand what his India has? I'm traveling here and giving up everything just to find it. And this guy thinks I'm *nuts?* I caught my internal rage. *Why am I so mean? How did I get so sarcastic and rude even while dressed as a sadhu? I'm such a freaking hypocrite! This guy is just shocked by a white sadhu. That's understandable.*

I tried to reason with my nasty attitude as the train rolled on, the monks chanted, and this guy gawked. I looked away from him and gazed out the window as if he hadn't asked me anything. I chanted on my mala.

Metal on metal was the music of the train. Occasionally, another train passed us going in the opposite direction. Still no air conditioning. All we had was the open window blowing hot air. My berth was still packed, even with only three to a bench. And I was still dealing with this new guy sitting across from me.

"Why, man?" he persisted.

How was I going to explain that material comforts won't satisfy the soul? His parents were probably religious, chanting on mala and worshiping deities. And his grandparents and great-grandparents most definitely. But this generation seemed to want something better. *Good luck with that*, I thought. They might have seen the images portrayed in Hollywood and magazines, but that was a dream. An apparition. They weren't seeing the back end. The twelve-step meetings from indulgence and addiction. The deforestation from raising cattle. The slaughterhouses. The overfed and undernourished obesity issues that come from too much fast food.

America's idea of a healthy meal at that time was eating a protein bar or drinking a shake. But there was no fast food in India in 1988. Even the poorest people in India ate fresh food every day. Made from scratch. They spiced it themselves. I had certainly never ground my own wheat berries to make fresh flour, but they did it all the time here. Nothing was frozen or processed. What had we traded for this illusive American dream? The quality of life. Sitting down and eating with a family. We'd lost out on high-quality living. We'd traded in homemade roti and butter for Costco tater tots and frozen french fries.

"Why, man?" he pressed.

I didn't answer him. He left to use the toilet. Another man, about fifty, well dressed and cultured, peered at me. He was wearing a wool vest with wooden buttons, handmade. Gandhi had supported this movement of creating your own fabrics, buttons, and soaps by hand with local ingredients. This man wore a dhoti and kurta, both made of khadi. He saw that I was disturbed by the young man's questioning.

"The boy is just curious," he said. "We have many sadhus in this country. But you are from a rich country. It is a rare thing to see. Where are you from?"

"Mai American hun," I said. "New York se hun." I tried my best to speak Hindi.

Thinking I was fluent, he started rattling off sentences as if I was a local. I had to interrupt him to say that I couldn't understand him.

"What is your good name?" he said, in staccato English.

I loved the way some people would say *good* name.

"Ray," I replied. "What is your name?"

"Bippin Sharma," he replied. He continued asking questions, but it was a sweet interrogation. "What was it like for you growing up in America? Why the life of a sadhu now?"

He genuinely wanted to know. So I told him, starting with my memories of high school.

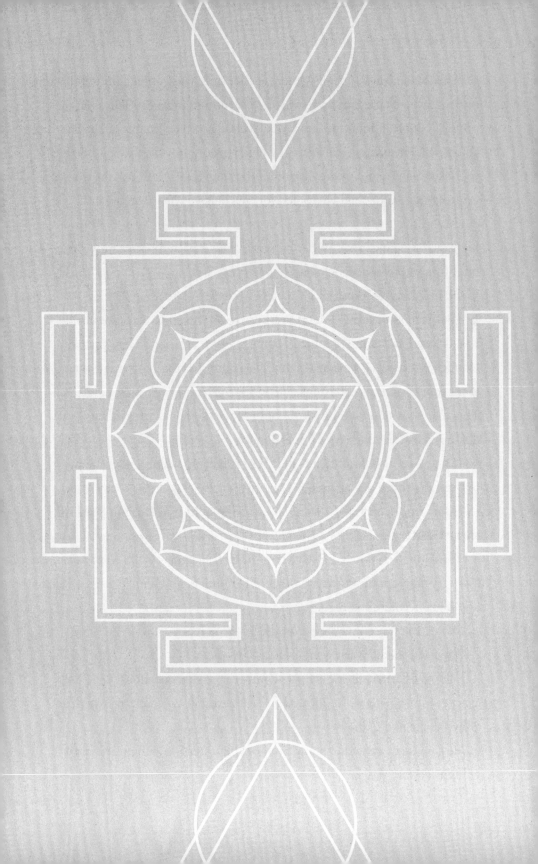

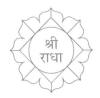

CHAPTER 2
HIGH SCHOOL & SPIRITUAL BEGINNINGS

My face was pushed against a locker. I was wearing combat boots and a beret with an X-Ray Spex button on it. My hair was cut into a faux hawk. I had on a vest that said "Hyperactive Child" across the back. Two kids, bigger than me, dressed in varsity jackets and flannel shirts, were crushing my head against a steel locker in a deserted hallway.

"What's up, Mr. Freak? You like being a freak, Mr. Freak? Is it fun for you?" They laughed as my cheekbone ground into the metal. I started drooling.

"Beats being a boring conformist," I said, pulling my head away from the locker.

They slammed it forward again, furious that I'd talked back to them.

"Yeah, how would you like these boring conformist guys to kick your ass, Mr. Freak?"

"Is that a trick question? Are you the dumbass brothers?" I acted fearless, but I was petrified. Before they could slam me into the locker for a third time, Mr. Cameron, the vice principal, walked around the corner.

"Mr. Cortez and Mr. Jameson," he said in a military voice. "Shouldn't you two be in class right now? And Mr. Cappo, don't you think you ask for this with the way you dress? It's provocative, and you know it."

"Yeah, he started it by dressing like a dork!" one of my aggressors said.

"You think I wanted this attention?" I said, peeling myself off the locker and straightening my clothes, looking squarely at the vice principal.

"If you want my honest opinion," he said, "yes, I think you want to stand out from the crowd and get some attention."

"Fortunately, I'm not interested in other people's opinions," I said softly, but firmly. "That would be a tragic way to live, wouldn't it, Mr. Cameron?"

"You're lucky your father is part of the faculty here, Mr. Cappo. Now, get to class."

Somehow, I was in trouble for getting jacked up against the locker. Fascinating.

That was why, every weekend, I escaped to New York City.

*　　*　　*

The kind Mr. Bippin Sharma listened attentively, so I continued. I loved talking to strangers. Especially on vehicles. They were trapped, and it became free therapy.

"I was in a band. A noisy sort of a band," I said. "Me and three friends, the high school freaks of my class. We had no real talent, but it was fun. We were called Violent Children."

Mr. Sharma furrowed his brow.

"It was just for shock value," I reassured him. "We weren't really violent. We were just kids, having fun, wanting to be different, trying to find ourselves in a culture where everyone looked the same and dressed the same. Our music came out of the frustration of living in a conformist suburb. Nobody listened to anything except mainstream music in our town. Boring arena rock bands."

Mr. Sharma nodded as if he understood the nuances of American culture—although I'm sure he didn't—so I didn't stop to explain anything.

* * *

In my hometown of Danbury, Connecticut, where the band and I went to high school, there was a university that had a college radio station. It was mainly boring corporate rock, but every Sunday night from 11 p.m. to 2 a.m., a DJ named Darryl would play all this avant-garde music that was impossible to hear on mainstream radio. He'd play punk, rockabilly, American hardcore, English punk rock, goth, electronic, and dance. It was great. This station, and other college radio stations with DJs like Darryl, were the only way to hear this type of music in much of the United States—and we only got a few hours a week. Eventually, these stations catalyzed an underground alternative music scene. My friends and I would stay up late to listen and call in requests. We all wanted to meet Darryl because people with a taste for the obscure were rare where we grew up. The punks, the outcasts, were a tiny demographic in Connecticut in 1982. A shaved head, mohawk, or combat boots were signs. You'd look them up and down to see if they were your punk or hardcore brethren or merely military guys. If they looked back at you and you made the connection, you'd realize they were one of you.

After Darryl's show, the radio station went right back to boring corporate rock again. AC/DC, Cheap Trick, Chicago, Ozzy, Jethro Tull. Darryl's slot, named *The Adventure Jukebox*, was an oasis and the highlight of our week. One weekend, we decided to bring Darryl our Violent Children demo tape. It was a long shot, since we didn't know him, but we thought maybe he'd play it on his show. We drove to the university late one night, right before he went on air.

None of the band drank or smoked. We all had peculiar haircuts and dressed slightly ridiculously. We wore absurd boots or Vans (which had to be special ordered at that time) and earrings. This was living on the edge in

1982. My father was repulsed when I showed up with my left ear pierced. He didn't even know what to say. I shrugged it off. *What other people think of me is none of my business. What I think of myself—that's my business.* A standard mantra in my teens.

All the doors at the radio station were locked. On the second story, we could see the DJ's studio with the lights on, even though everything else was turned off. The cold November air cut through my parachute pants and army jacket. We got pebbles from the parking lot and started throwing them at the window. After the fourth pebble, a spry elf of a man with a Fun Boy Three hairdo appeared. It was Darryl.

"What's up? What do you guys want?"

"We're in a local hardcore band, and we have a demo we want you to play," I said.

He got excited and said he'd send somebody right down. We were all escorted up to the studio, feeling like royalty. In hindsight, that demo was a piece of crap. None of us could play our instruments. It had been recorded with a boom box in my parents' two-car garage.

"I can't believe there's a band from Danbury!" he said when we got up there. "Of course I'll play your demo!"

The song he was spinning stopped. The ON AIR light went on, and he put his finger to his lips. "We have very special guests *live* in the studio," he said in his crisp DJ voice. "Danbury's own Violent Children! Yes, Violent Children are here in the studio with their very first demo, which we're going to showcase tonight!"

He went on praising us, as if we were talented. Then he played the song. Afterward, he spoke highly of it to both the listeners and to us privately. The phone started ringing. Darryl picked up, then handed me the receiver. "This is a guy from New York City. He says he wants to book Violent Children at A7."

I was shocked. New York City? At A7, one of the coolest underground after-hours clubs in the city? We'd never played a gig in our lives.

Then another call came through. "This guy is from Stamford," said Darryl. "He wants to book you at Pogo's in Bridgeport." Pogo's was the biggest punk club in Connecticut.

"I think we just got our big break," my bass player said. "This is unbelievable!"

The promoter at Pogo's called me Monday morning. I knew about the club because it advertised shows in the back of local newspapers. Bands like Black Flag, Flipper, the Circle Jerks. Massive California bands that were touring the nation.

"My name's Brian. I run an art gallery and underground club in Stamford called the Anthrax," he said. "It was recently shut down, so we're doing a benefit at Pogo's and would love for you guys to play. I could introduce you to everyone. Connecticut's got a great underground music and art scene. Not sure if you're aware of that."

I held the receiver and just sort of nodded. "I go to New York for shows and art. I didn't really think anything happened in Connecticut." In truth, I had never been to a gallery in my life. I didn't know that New York City street art was taking off and that his gallery promoted it.

"Connecticut is incredible!" he insisted. "Look, we got gear, just bring your guitars and a snare drum to Pogo's on Saturday night. You're going on second. We got a bunch of bands playing—Agnostic Front, Hose, Urban Waste, Reagan Youth, the Vatican Commandos—it's going to be huge. Get here for 8 p.m."

The following week, I asked my dad if we could borrow his Volkswagen Rabbit and drive to Bridgeport for a gig. He was incredibly trusting of me, even though the previous year I had slam danced a giant hole in the supporting wall of our living room during a punk party I threw while my parents were in Italy. I'd tried my best to patch, plaster, and paint it, but they'd figured it out. I was humiliated.

I was the second youngest out of seven kids, and none of my siblings appreciated the punk/freak stage I was in. Not one bit. But my dad was tolerant, and we loaded up that compact car with guitars and a snare and headed to Bridgeport, which was fifty minutes away. I had never left my hometown, except for the occasional field trip, and this was the beginning of forty years of traveling the world.

As we pulled up, night was falling. We saw an older guy with a bright-blue spiked mohawk, Converse shoes, and a buttoned-up shirt. There were gangs of people wearing leather jackets with band names and slogans painted on their backs. Freaks, weird haircuts, young kids smoking cigarettes, piercings, Doc Martens, and creepers.

My people! I thought. Still, an element of fear blended with the excitement. I was a little intimidated to get out of the car. We gathered our gear and politely strutted to the front door.

"We're in Violent Children," I said to the burly bouncer taking money.

A slick, leather-jacket-wearing twentysomething with sharp cheekbones and engineer boots spoke up. "Are you Ray? I'm Brian. Welcome to Pogo's. Come on in."

In retrospect, I don't think Brian was more than ten years older than me. But when you're sixteen, anyone who's fully grown seems like a man. And he wore cologne.

"This is Jeff Cud, *Connecticut Underground Dispatch,*" he told us. "It's a local music magazine. And this is Moby and Chuck Wheat, from the Vatican Commandos."

We all nodded and pushed through the crowd.

"If you ever want to play in Utah, here's the guy to talk to," Brian said, pointing to a man in a brown leather jacket who gave me a nod and shook my hand.

The club was noisy and packed with weirdos, including punk-looking girls, who I never saw in my high school, wearing short leopard-print dresses, high boots, and spiked hair. Although I was drawn to this alternative world, the smell of the smoke and beer was nauseating, and I was honestly a little let down. Our band didn't drink alcohol or smoke cigarettes or marijuana. We rebelled against all that. It seemed foolish. Sit around a keg. Get drunk. Act stupid. In one sense, I thought this music scene was an alternative oasis, but on the other, all these adults were heavily drinking and smoking—worse than the people I knew in high school. This bothered me. But I moved forward because I admired the nonconformity and DIY ethics of the scene. I loved that these kids were making their own music, as primitive as it was, instead of covering someone else's music, a poor imitation of the arena rock bands. It was original. Fresh. Energetic. And it was raw. To be punk or hardcore was to be bold in a world that scoffed at you.

We were second on the bill, slotted to play a thirty-minute set, with seven or so bands playing after us, including some that I already loved, like Reagan Youth, Urban Waste, and Agnostic Front. We got on the stage and played nervously, but the community was supportive. The crowd cheered and stage dived for our set.

Being on stage was the greatest thrill of my life. At that point I was the drummer. I *loved* the drums. It was exhausting and wonderful, but I envied the singer. I always felt like a front man.

After the show, people started circling us to talk. Old people, young people, *girls*. I had never had this kind of dopamine hit from being admired so much—and for doing relatively little. After we'd been chatting for a while and collecting some phone numbers, Brian suddenly ran toward us.

"The cops are here," he said. "We're getting raided. I need all you kids under twenty-one to get under the stage and hide! Now! There's a little door you can climb into."

None of us were over seventeen. The stage was only about eighteen inches high. We moved quickly, getting on our hands and knees. We were covered in dirt and dust and spider webs, and it was pitch black. I was too excited to be freaked out. I heard cops yelling and people running around above me. I heard sirens outside the door. *If I get thrown in a Bridgeport prison tonight, my father is going to kill me*, I thought.

41

After an hour under the stage, bands started playing again over our heads. It sounded like things were back to normal. We waited another thirty minutes, then snuck out and reintegrated with the people in the club. The cops were gone. One thing was for sure, this was worlds away from my suburban high school life.

We stayed to watch some more bands, and I walked outside between sets. An older guy in a black leather jacket, ripped black jeans, and motorcycle boots came up to me. "My name's Johnny, and I got a club in the city where you could play," he said in a New York accent. "I talked to you on the phone the other day at the radio station. Would you kids be into it?"

I nodded, trying to be cool. I had been to his club, A7, a few times. For this type of music, A7 was a holy place where every cool underground band played. It was on the southwest corner of Tompkins Square Park—also known as Needle Park, as it was filled with junkies day and night. It was a lawless time in a lawless neighborhood. It was an illegal after-hours bar, operating from midnight to 5 a.m. on the weekends without a liquor license at an especially corrupt time in New York City history. There was no sign. You just had to know where it was. Outside of the entrance door was a menacing, spray-painted warning: "Out of Town Bands, Realize Where You Are."

Danger was an aroma always in the air on the Lower East Side, and to be in that neighborhood after midnight was a risk, especially if you were only sixteen. For me, watching bands and hanging out there on weekends was like visiting the Wild West in the time of Jesse James and John Wesley Hardin. There were junky zombies, anarchists, nonconformists, squatters, and gangs. And violent crime was normalized by the punks in the scene, neighborhood kids who didn't like outsiders, and out-of-control drunks or addicts. Anything could happen, and it usually did. We were forced to learn street smarts quick.

I'd been going to New York City on my own since I was fourteen, telling my parents almost every weekend that I was "going to watch music."

They must have thought I was going to the Philharmonic or something because they encouraged me, never knowing the danger I willingly placed myself in each week. I'd take the train back Sunday evening and show up for school on Monday. My classmates could never imagine the things I had seen or done from Friday to Sunday.

But I fit in there. I loved it. And A7 was at the heart of that turbulent chaos, drawing me like iron to a magnet, despite the fear.

"I got a show coming up in February if you want to get on that," Johnny said.

"Ah, sure we'll take it," I said.

It was at A7 that I met Harley Flanagan, notorious leader of the new band Cro-Mags. He befriended me one night and would influence my future in ways I could not have imagined at the time. You never know who God's going to send to you to deliver a noble message of truth.

Believe it or not, Harley Flanagan was my first unofficial guru.

*　*　*

I followed Harley down Bleecker Street. He'd seen me standing outside CBGB during a Sunday matinee between bands and invited me on a walk. He deftly spun a chair leg in his hand like a baton. It had a little nail sticking out of it, making it a gnarly weapon. He could have easily decided to swing it at my shaven skull for no good reason, and nobody would have seen or cared. He'd used this weapon on the unsuspecting before. But I was in good standing with him, as far as I knew. Other people knew it, too, and didn't mess with me. I partly credit Harley for my protection on the Lower East Side.

Still, he was marching me down the street, running off at the mouth about what I later realized was transcendental wisdom, Vedic knowledge, and the *Bhagavad Gita*. I shut up and listened. Although he was a year younger than me, it seemed like he'd lived lifetimes. His band had started as a street gang.

Sonically, they were incredible and fierce, the kind of music I liked, with a message that appealed to my sinister side. I was a teenager trying to figure out who I was. He was already a legend in the punk scene and a gifted musician. In sixth grade, when most kids are still in Cub Scouts, he was playing drums for a New York City punk band. Not even old enough to grow a mustache, he had rubbed elbows with Deborah Harry of Blondie, Joe Strummer of the Clash, and Andy Warhol. He even wrote a book with Allen Ginsberg.

That was his artistic side. But he was also hotheaded and could turn on someone in a moment. I both feared him and looked up to him. I felt elite and important that this young celebrity was even noticing me. I was a nobody, a sheltered kid with little life experience, and this guy gave me clout just by talking to me. I was also freaked out because of his propensity for unpredictability and violence. Controversy followed him everywhere.

I knew he hung out with Krishnas, who blended into the Lower East Side tapestry with their freakish outfits and chanting. I didn't get it. But I was somewhat aware that the Vedic teachings of the Krishnas serendipitously had opened Harley's world and inspired his lyrics, song titles, and record covers—and I admired his artistry.

I started to feel vulnerable, but I followed Harley down the decrepit subway stairs to an empty station that reeked of urine. He was still spouting philosophical concepts similar to those of Mahatma Gandhi, while I tried to figure out where his ideals met reality. I didn't know whether he was divine or demonic, and at that time, he might not have known either. But I hadn't heard these concepts before: "Spirit is eternal and always reincarnating." "Religion is one. God is one. All these different paths are meant to bring you to surrender to God." "We don't have a soul; we are a soul and we have a body." "Even animals are spiritual beings. Even trees and plants. They are all spirit souls, just wearing different outfits."

I was impressed and nodded along, taking care not to look at him wrong. Truthfully, I'd never thought about such deep philosophical concepts, but

I began to appreciate the paradigm-shifting ideas he was talking about. It resonated somewhere deep in my heart of hearts. He'd had enough of talking to me and invited me to jump on the subway to Brooklyn to go to the Krishna temple for a Sunday feast and *Bhagavad Gita* class. My mom was from Brooklyn, and she'd told me, "Brooklyn's off limits. It's too dangerous." Harley seemed too dangerous, too. So I politely refused.

He slapped my hand in a gesture of friendship, looked the token booth man in the eye, and hopped the turnstile. The man began yelling through the intercom in a muffled voice, "Get back here. Officer, hurry. White T-shirt coming down, Brooklyn bound." Of course, no cops responded, so Harley turned around, calmly faced the attendant, and flipped him off.

This was my introduction to Vedic thought and the bhakti tradition. Not through a swami, sage, hermit, or guru, but through a teenage gang member and part-time transcendentalist. Truthfully, if I'd run into a proper guru at the time—an actual spiritual teacher—I wouldn't have given him the time of day. Truth had to be delivered in this particular package. The universe chooses perfect messengers for us when we become seekers.

* * *

My growing sensitivity to violence and suffering had also made me want to change our band name. I'd grown to hate the moniker Violent Children. It was stupid. I wasn't violent and didn't want to promote violence. I'd picked the name Violent Children for shock value. It had worked, but I'd grown out of it quickly. I *was* violent in junior high school. I was bullied, stolen from, on the receiving end of regular humiliation. So I lifted weights, learned how to box, and randomly picked fights for no good reason except to establish myself as the bully and not the bullied. That incarnation of myself had lasted about a year and a half; then punk and hardcore had given me other things to think about and relate to: peace, unity, open-mindedness, and positivity. At the same time, violence pervaded the scene, and I didn't want to be on the receiving end of some Lower East Side beatdown. I was confused. I didn't know if I was a pacifist, an anarchist, or something else. So I tried to stay neutral and under the radar in the city. I wasn't ready to stake any claim.

As I grew up, I realized I wanted the music I wrote to uplift the world, not degrade the world. I liked the concept of DIY. Like pretty much everyone else in the scene, my band and I did everything ourselves. We created our own music, booked our own shows, made our own magazines, started our own record labels, and booked our own tours. But did I have to opt in to the dark side that came with that hardcore punk package? I hoped not.

Things changed when I fell in love with a band from Reno, Nevada, called 7 Seconds. Whether he knew it or not, Kevin Seconds, the singer and songwriter, became my first teacher. Not a guru, like Harley Flanagan, but the first person I saw who showed me that you could be part of the scene without opting into all the negativity of the punk ethos. His songs checked all the boxes of the music I loved: they were fast, furious, raw, heartfelt, distorted, and powerful, but they also had lyrics that made it okay to be vulnerable, kind, loving, and self-disciplined. This was a colossal shift in a punk scene riddled with toxic thinking, reactionary finger pointing, and degrading habits that led to addiction and suicide.

Around the same time, the guitar player of Violent Children—my teenage best friend, John "Porcell" Porcelly—and I decided to start a new band, rebrand ourselves, and claim new identities. Although they didn't know it, 7 Seconds gave us the permission to stand up for the things that we believed in, even when the majority of our scene did not.

We called the band Youth of Today, and our mission was simple: make the most furious sounding music and use it to bring epic change to ourselves and the world. We wanted to spread a message of clean living, self-discipline, and a positive mental attitude. Porcell was a skilled guitarist, and I finally got to be the singer, leaving my drumsticks behind. Two of

Porcell's friends joined the band on bass and drums, and we immediately started making waves and booking gigs.

We rallied behind the straight-edge label, which had been coined a couple of years earlier by Ian MacKaye of Minor Threat. Although Ian had never meant for straight edge to be a movement, I picked up the ball and ran with it. If Ian was Jesus, I was probably Matthew or Paul, as one podcaster later described me. I strongly felt that our world was crumbling before our eyes, and it couldn't hurt to broadcast the importance of positivity and abstinence. I rarely drank alcohol, but I'd witnessed the addiction, foolish behavior, and self-destruction caused by it. Same with drugs. There was no romance there for me. I wanted to represent an alternative: self-change. No more blaming. I led by example.

I may have saved my own life. And over the years, I've heard from many fans that these principles helped save theirs as well. We, somewhat unintentionally, upcycled Ian's term *straight edge* and helped it become an international movement—a positive subculture within the nihilistic scene of American punk and hardcore music.

*   *   *

In 1985 I moved to New Haven, Connecticut, to a house filled with Yalies. I was going to Southern Connecticut State University and studying math. But all I wanted to do was take my band on the road and tour. Still, I was in good company in New Haven. I had a solid crew of punkers, including my introverted high school friend Jordan Cooper, who was going to school there, too.

I wanted to see the world, meet people, and sing our songs. Maybe release a record or two. Promote positive change. I knew I wouldn't last in university. I quickly realized that, for most people, going to college was less about learning and more about partying and one-night stands. I felt above it. Over it. Trying to fit into a broken world was an unattractive and repulsive prospect. I wanted to contribute, which seemed a more noble pursuit than studying advanced calculus. I knew I had a bigger calling, and I needed like-minded friends. As I skateboarded around campus, I found a sign advertising a Christian club. I thought this might be a good group to connect with, and that it could shield me from the insanity of the university social scene. I hadn't been to a church since childhood, but I accepted the teachings as sacred and considered myself more spiritual than religious.

I skated into that meeting wearing bleached blond hair, an earring, a bandana around my head, and a black sleeveless vest. The other Christians in the club seemed conservative and normal. *Real* normal. I was okay with that. I liked dressing differently, but I didn't look down upon those who were straitlaced.

We read from Matthew 18:21–22 that night: "Then Peter came to Jesus and asked, 'Lord, how many times shall I forgive my brother or sister who sins against me? Up to seven times?' Jesus answered, 'I tell you, not seven times, but seventy-seven times.'"

Then from Luke 6:37: "Do not judge, and you will not be judged. Do not condemn, and you will not be condemned. Forgive, and you will be forgiven."

I loved this. I started reading the New Testament and appreciating it in a new way. These concepts of compassion, forgiveness, salvation for social outcasts, and a deep faith in a higher benevolent force spoke to me and blended well with my philosophy of positive living and trusting the universe.

I felt like I had found a home and that I was learning deep truths. Jesus was dedicated to feeding the hungry, healing the sick, and commissioning his followers to bring God into the world, despite public opposition. The other group members and I practiced this in our own community. For example, we went to hospitals to provide comfort to the elderly. This feeling of giving to those in need offered deep internal joy.

Although I enjoyed the meetings, support, and camaraderie, I started questioning the exclusivity of the teachings. *What about Jews? Muslims? Hindus?*

Where do they fit in with the bigger picture of connecting with God? I thought. I noticed that there was an underlying sentiment among the group that other faith traditions were not only excluded from spiritual experiences but also stemmed from a malevolent force that misled, misguided, and ultimately imprisoned their followers' eternal souls. I found this difficult to swallow.

While I studied the New Testament, I also discovered another book that fascinated me called the *Dhammapada*, a collection of sayings of the Buddha in verse form. The name *Dhammapada* literally translates to "at the feet of dharma." I sat in my room, burned some nag champa incense, and read a passage from the chapter titled "The Thousands":

> Better than a thousand useless words is one useful
> word, hearing which one attains peace.
>
> Better than a thousand useless verses is one useful
> verse, hearing which one attains peace.
>
> Better than reciting a hundred meaningless verses
> is reciting one verse of Dhamma, hearing which
> one attains peace.
>
> Though one may conquer a thousand times a
> thousand men in battle, yet he indeed is the
> noblest victor who conquers himself.
>
> Self-conquest is far better than the conquest
> of others. Not even a god, an angel, Mara [death]
> or Brahma can turn into defeat the victory of such
> a person who is self-subdued and ever restrained
> in conduct.

I was excited to share the words of the Buddha with my Christian friends at the next meeting, especially since these teachings seemed so Christlike.

After the opening prayers, we went around the room checking in with each other. When it was my turn to speak, I lit up.

"You know how I like wisdom literature and progressive living?" I asked. "Well, I found this book that I think you guys will like. It's Buddhist and seems to go hand in hand with everything Jesus taught in the New Testament."

I reached into my backpack, opened the *Dhammapada* to a marked page in the chapter called "Violence," and read the following:

> All tremble at violence. Life is dear to all. Putting oneself in the place of another, one should not kill nor cause another to kill.
>
> One who while himself seeking happiness oppresses with violence other beings who also desire happiness, will not attain happiness hereafter.

I looked up and saw cynical, scornful glances. I was confused.

Glenn, the elected leader of the group, and perhaps the most biblically astute, was the first to speak. "Ray, these books can *appear* deep or thoughtful, but you have to be careful with them. They can also be very misleading." Another group member started to condemn me, but Glenn quickly cut him down. "I'm not saying it's bad. Just misleading. We're going to stick to the Bible here."

I felt a little muzzled and minimized, and my punk attitude of rebellion started to get stirred up, but I sat there in silence. After all, it was a Bible study group. Perhaps I'd been out of line.

The next person in the circle was a guy named Oliver. Instead of sharing his life, his struggles, or his successes, he started picking apart what I'd shared. "I'm so glad Glenn shut down the reading of that book," he said. "I don't want to even *hear* words from the Buddha. If you imagine how many people Satan has misled with these doctrines, it's heartbreaking." He looked around dramatically.

"Have you even read this book?" I asked, out of turn.

"No," he snapped. "I don't have to eat dirt to know I don't like it."

"Well, that's your loss. You're missing out." I looked him dead in the eyes. "It could even help you get closer to Jesus."

"Ray, these books aren't going to help you on your spiritual quest," Oliver said. "They're going to send you straight to hell."

"Why?" I asked. "Did you hear what I was reading? How is that any different from what Jesus says in the New Testament? In my opinion, a lot of the world's problems come from seeing the differences in people, religions, or political parties. The more you look for differences, the more you find them. Why not look for the commonalities? It would be a much more beautiful world than what you're suggesting."

Oliver made a disgusted face, so I turned to Glenn, who seemed more reasonable and mature. "Glenn," I said earnestly, "where would *you* say a good Buddhist goes when they die? A good Buddhist, who follows all the teachings of their path? One who develops compassion, love, sensitivity to others, conquers their senses. Where would they go?"

"It's very clearly stated in the Bible," said another member, who I didn't know. "'I am the way, the truth, and the life. No one comes to the Father except through Me.'"

"What more do you need to hear, Ray?" asked Oliver. "Jesus said it himself."

"The Buddha says similar things," I replied. "'Nobody can cross the great ocean except through Me.' Maybe Christ meant without a teacher, or a guru, nobody can understand—"

Once I said "guru," it seemed like they all turned against me.

"Jesus wasn't a guru, Ray, he was God!" Glenn said.

"Well if he was God," I shot back, "why did he say, 'No one comes to the Father except through Me'? He's distinguishing between Himself and God. Or 'I'm seated at the right hand of the Father.' I'll ask again, where would that good, sincere Buddhist go in your opinion, Glenn?"

Glenn pursed his lips and closed his eyes, as if hoping for divine intervention. But he didn't answer.

"Where?"

"He's going to hell, Ray."

"What?" I was dumbfounded. "Because somebody was born in a different culture, before there was global transportation, and strictly followed all the rules of their spiritual heritage and perhaps never met a Christian, they are doomed to hell? Eternally?"

"Yes!" said Oliver.

"How is that even fair?" I asked. "What if you were born before Christ was alive? All of these millions of souls are condemned because they were born at the wrong time? They never even had the opportunity to meet Christ! They're all going to hell?" I was devastated and disturbed.

Glenn nodded.

"What about John the Baptist, Abraham, and every good Jew who followed all 613 commandments? What about Moses?" I asked, my voice rising. "They're *all* going to suffer eternally? Do you hear how ludicrous that sounds? What kind of a sadistic God do you believe in? That's not an all-loving God. That's a barbaric God. Why would an all-loving God make His children suffer"—I paused, drawing the next word out slowly—"*eternally*? Just because they were born at the wrong time or in the wrong place? I don't buy it!"

Glenn tried to regain his composure and take back control of the meeting. "Let's just continue with our circle of sharing before we do our reading," he said. "These are all great questions, Ray."

I felt patronized. If they were great questions, why didn't anyone have great answers? They all just shut me down.

After the sharing, we read about the resurrection of Christ. The mood in the room had relaxed again.

I raised my hand. "Do you ever wonder what you do in heaven?" I asked the room. "And who goes? Is it a five-year-old version of me? Or an old version of me? Do I get a new body? One without aches and pains and wrinkles? Will my grandfather who died in his eighties have a child's body? Do we meet relatives?"

No answer.

I persisted. "Who are the demons that Christ exorcised? Are they like bad angels? Are they fully bad or just confused ghosts?"

Nobody answered. They may have thought I was being ridiculous or sarcastic. But I wasn't. I wanted to see if they'd ever thought about these things.

"What about animals? Do dogs go to heaven when they die?"

"Any other questions?" Glenn asked, without addressing any of mine.

I raised my hand and spoke simultaneously. "The way that you reject all other paths except your own . . . I find it shocking. I don't get this when I read the Bible. I feel like I'm reading a different book than you are."

I packed up my things and left in a fluster, never to return. I was so upset. This group had been an oasis for me. I never told the band or my punk friends in New Haven about my Christian dabbling. I thought they wouldn't understand. But the more I studied wisdom literature from different spiritual traditions, the deeper my lyrics became—and, of course, I realized how much the different spiritual traditions had in common.

* * *

Thanksgiving 1985 seemed like a typical family gathering, something we did on the major holidays. Come back from wherever we were in the world and gather. Talk our shit. Fight a little. Catch each other up. Eat a lot. Laugh a lot. Give unsolicited advice. Exchange some presents. Show some special love to Mom and Dad. And find some commonality among siblings who were different and who had big Italian mouths and egos.

Mom had told us that Dad had a cold, but when I arrived, she said that he was in the hospital. Then we got a message that he was in critical condition in the ICU. All seven of us kids stayed on the phone extensions peppered around our mom's house, listening to the doctor speak in a grave voice. He told all of us that our father was *not* going to make it through the night. I had never heard my older brothers cry, but we all cried that night. I stood in disbelief. How? What had happened? (We found out later that it was some type of lung infection, but he never received a proper diagnosis.)

One of my older sisters tried to be a rock in the storm. "We have to pull together," she said after we hung up with the doctor.

I walked outside into the falling snow. *Pull together?* I thought. *Why?* A sniper called Death was picking us off for no good reason. He didn't care that it was a holiday.

I was devastated by the randomness. The bad timing. Thanksgiving night. What had my honest, hardworking father ever done to deserve this? I started sobbing into my hands, walking aimlessly, not dressed for snow. By coincidence, I had been reading *On Death and Dying* by Elisabeth Kübler-Ross. I had the book with me, opened it up, and read this quote:

> It's only when we truly know and understand that
> we have a limited time on earth—and that we have
> no way of knowing when our time is up, we will then
> begin to live each day to the fullest, as if it was the
> only one we had.

My father ended up making it through the night. We crowded around his bed until they told us we had to leave. The doctors said he was coming out of it. We were all shaken, but they convinced us to calm down and go home. He remained in a room at the hospital, which seemed desolate and depressing for a place of healing. It reeked of broken hearts, bitterness, and sad memories from all those times when the sniper had hit his mark.

My misfortune caused me to turn inward. Wasn't Dad's random encounter with death *my* random encounter? I wasn't going to be spared either.

The hospital patients were just a few steps ahead of me in line. I kept returning to the Kübler-Ross quote. I realized that the real question wasn't about when I was going to die. It was about what I was supposed to do while I was living. Where was I going? What did I want?

My father was born in obscurity in Jamaica, Queens, the youngest of eleven from first-generation Italian immigrants during the Great Depression. His father died when my dad was only five. He was raised by his mom, who I never really knew. He and his brother, eighteen and twenty, were drafted by the army to fight in World War II. His brother was killed. Dad got his master's at New York University and married his first girlfriend (my mother) after three months of courtship. He became an English teacher and guidance counselor and was religious, honorable, and dutiful. He worked his way up through the public school system, retired, and a year later . . . he was in the hospital.

Were we here just to be good? Have a few adventures? Educate ourselves and pop out some kids? Was that a home run? Should we collect and consume as much stuff as we could? Or should we live life as a sacrifice to others, like Mother Teresa? Was it better to be as reckless as we could because we only live once? To act on any desire or whim that came to our mind? Or should we wander, trying to put our feet on every continent of the world? Should we gather knowledge, learn languages, heal people, fight for causes? What the hell were we doing here? And were we feebly creating meaning when perhaps there was no meaning whatsoever?

While dad stayed at the hospital, we were supposed to enjoy Thanksgiving. Before my dad's health scare, my main concern was breaking the news to my family that I had become a vegetarian. I still had to do it, and I knew they wouldn't take it lightly. Meat was a staple in our Italian American household. My parents had grown up during the Depression, and in their view, only the poorest of the poor were vegetarian. It was a symbol of hard work to afford meat. My vegetarianism would be a slap in the face to our father.

At this point in time, vegetarianism and veganism weren't part of mainstream conversation and were reserved for people my family would likely describe as hippie, granola-eating tree huggers. But in high school, I had read the 1975 classic *Animal Liberation: A New Ethics for Our Treatment of Animals* by Peter Singer, and it struck a chord with me. It took me many more years to digest its message and to try to put it into practice. Which is what I was doing that Thanksgiving.

I won't lie—it was difficult. I loved eating meat, and there weren't a lot of resources out there. You couldn't just go out and buy a veggie burger. I didn't know any vegetarians, and I didn't know how to cook anything. But as soon as I turned eighteen and started living on my own, I decided that I was going to minimize the violence in my life, starting with everything I could control, like my meals. I gave up all meat except fish.

During Thanksgiving dinner, I made an announcement: "Attention everyone. I've become a vegetarian. I'm not going to eat turkey this year. I find it ethically abominable." I tried to be colorful and dramatic. Most of my siblings didn't even look up. They just kept eating.

"Did anyone hear what Ray said?" my brother asked. "He thinks it's ethically wrong to eat a bird that's bred to be eaten. It was made to be food. Whatever. More for us."

"Ray, you'll die if you don't eat meat," said my mother. "Don't be a fool. You need protein. You're gonna become skinny and malnourished. Who's teaching you this?"

"Who cares what he eats?" said someone else. "Let him eat whatever he wants to. He's a grown man now."

"We are all spiritual beings," I said. "If I'm going to extend love and affection to a dog or a cat, why wouldn't I do that to a pig or a cow?" That got their attention. Forks and knives were placed on the table.

"Because they're *pigs* and *cows*."

"Don't you understand that there's no difference?" I defended myself.

"There's a *tremendous* difference," my brother argued. "They're not dogs, they're cows. We eat cows. We don't eat dogs."

We went back and forth a bit longer. They didn't quite understand me, but they sensed my sincerity. Thanksgiving carried on. I never ended up telling my father. He never left the hospital, and he died three years later.

*   *   *

Magic happened one day in late 1985. 7 Seconds asked us to join their West Coast tour, which coincided with winter break, and offered to put out our newly recorded album on their new label, Positive Force. It was like winning the lottery! I had met them a year earlier on their first East Coast tour, and we'd become friends. 7 Seconds was an internationally beloved band, and they were signing us, believing in us, and inviting us to tour with them. I felt like my positive choices were putting me where I wanted to be in life. All of this confirmed my convictions that we were doing something good for the world. The universe was reciprocating.

I reached out to my mother to check on my father. She said he was on the road to recovery. Over the years, his illness had its ups and downs. But at that time, this news gave me hope. Everything was looking up. But then, three days before we were scheduled to leave for the tour, our drummer announced that he'd never bought his plane ticket and didn't want to go. We were shocked. I was devastated. Broken. Shattered.

When I called Kevin Seconds, he told us to come out as planned and that they would find us a drummer. He reassured me that we'd have a few days to practice before the first gig. Kevin was laid back. Not worried. Down to earth. I loved him for that. So I trusted it would work out as the universe intended it to.

Nothing was very professional about our tour. We were on the punk/hardcore circuit, and that meant most of it was DIY. We flew into Reno and drove to the practice studio, which was nothing more than a rented storage unit where the band practiced illegally. When I asked Kevin about our drummer, he nonchalantly said that he would do it.

"But I probably won't remember all the songs on such short notice," he added. "So I'll play the first half of the set, and Troy, our drummer, will play the other half."

"Do you even play drums?" I asked, amazed and a little skeptical.

"Sort of. It'll be good. It'll work out."

That was why I loved punk. Kevin believed in what we were doing, and that positivity and love was louder than musical perfection. The attitude was contagious. I felt honored to have my teenage hero as my touring drummer.

Practice went well, and the rest of 7 Seconds and their roadies showed up in a 1971 Chevy passenger van that had seen better days. As crappy and small as the van was, it looked like a luxury tour bus to me.

"This is what we're touring in?" I asked excitedly.

"No, that's *my* band's van," Kevin said, a little embarrassed. "We won't all fit. I'm driving you guys in another vehicle."

Right on cue, Troy pulled up in a wreck of a car—a 1972 Ford station wagon with no license plates.

"Can this car make it up and down California and Arizona?" Porcell asked in disbelief.

"Ah, it'll probably be okay." Kevin wasn't as convincing this time. I asked about the license plates and registration. "We'll find plates," he said. "I think we have some somewhere."

Our fate was in the hands of forces greater than ourselves, and Porcell and I loved it. He looked at me and said, "It's all gonna work out." And it did. It always did.

I got to meet every West Coast punk celebrity and junior celebrity on that tour. We played our third show in front of three thousand people at Fender's Ballroom in Long Beach, California. We skateboarded with

Pushead, the graphic artist, and hung out with bands like Social Distortion, the Vandals, D.I., Doggy Style, and Uniform Choice, as well as *Maximum Rocknroll* editor Tim Yohannan, Fat Mike from NOFX, and Jello Biafra of Dead Kennedys.

Touring and spreading our message in our corner of the world may have been a small action, but it was something I could do that had a tangible effect. We were making it cool to be teenagers that didn't drink, smoke, or eat meat. I never went back to university after the tour, even though the rest of the band did. I had found my calling. I just wanted to be in a band, make music, tour, put out records, and spread our positive message. I stayed for a few months after the tour with 7 Seconds, living obligation-free. I hiked the Grand Canyon, camped, and drove to LA to pick up boxes of our new EP, *Can't Close My Eyes*. It was like the birth of a child. It helped us rise to new heights in the music scene and opened previously closed doors. We were in the flow, and everything was working out as if by magic. Everything felt like it was at our fingertips.

After the record was released, I went back to Connecticut to visit my father, who I'd thought was recovering. But while I was gone, his lungs had collapsed, leaving him comatose. My mother visited the hospital every day, and my siblings each reacted differently. I went to visit him, too, but I felt hopeless. His eyes moved as if he were looking at me, but the doctors said they weren't sure he could hear anything I said. I dealt with the tragedy by not dealing with it. I couldn't. Those big questions—about the purpose and meaning of life—would start creeping back into my consciousness, and I wasn't ready to face them.

So I let myself be numb. I turned off my emotions. If I had left them on, I think they would have crushed me. I left to start my life in New York City. I left my mother and siblings to sort out my father's condition. Hospital care. Insurance. Medical bills. Deductibles. Meetings with doctors.

I hoped things might turn around for him. They never did.

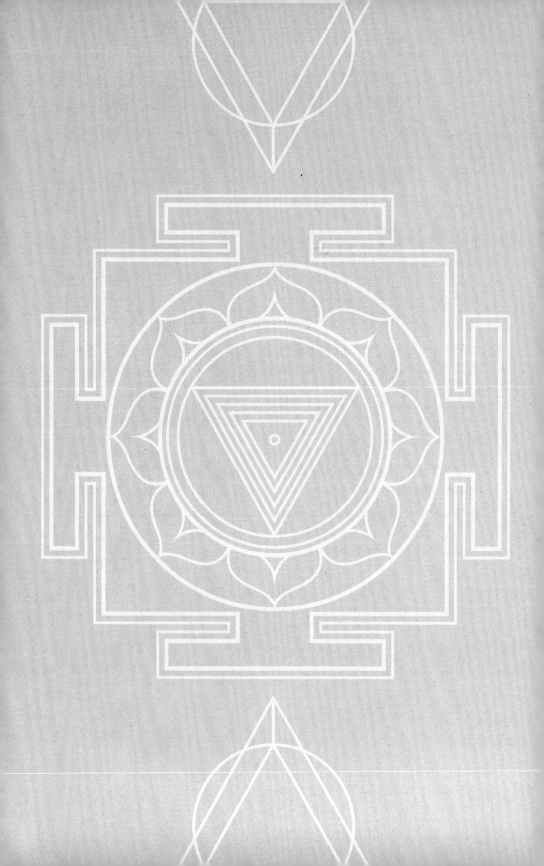

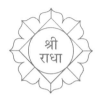

CHAPTER 3

NYC, THE BIRTH OF STRAIGHT EDGE & GROWING CONVICTIONS

My family had a rent-stabilized apartment in New York City that had been passed down through my brothers and sisters. It was on West Fifteenth Street and Eighth Avenue, which at that time was a disinvested, predominately Latinx area. It was an old tenement. Nothing fancy. The bathtub was in the kitchen, and the toilet, although private, was in the hallway in a closet. It was a railroad flat, as they were called—a studio apartment that had a small living room, kitchen, and bedroom all in a row like railway cars. No privacy from room to room, since there were no doors. There was no sunlight either, since it was on the ground floor and the windows faced a three-story wall. But the rent was $248 a month, heat included. That was going to be cut in half when Porcell moved in, as he'd promised he would after the latest semester at SUNY Oswego was over.

It was 1986, a great cultural moment to be in New York City: There was the rise of hip-hop, cool graffiti and street art, and a vibrant break-dancing scene. Madonna and KRS-One walked the streets, and the Beastie Boys were blowing up. Punk was becoming metal and metal was becoming punk. The cops were corrupt, and the streets were lawless, which made the underground culture flourish. The Lower East Side was still full of outcasts, freaks, artists, and seekers. And I was about to become part of an enormous straight-edge movement that would sweep the city and the world.

Two of our band members quit to pursue professional careers, but Porcell and I wanted this. I began actively searching for a new drummer and bass player. I found two sixteen-year-olds, Tommy and Craig, to play drums and bass. Both were incredible musicians, and Craig went on to tour the world with the hardcore punk band Sick of It All.

*   *   *

As New York City punk and hardcore music started blending with faster forms of heavy metal, Porcell and I began moving away from it. We found the metal scene cheesy and vapid. We felt that it was more about image than substance. But the world *needed* substance.

The books I read continued to influence my lyrics and attitudes. I liked spiritual and self-help books because I felt their time-tested messages could help me have the greatest impact on my audience. As David J. Schwartz wrote in *The Magic of Thinking Big*, "Believe it can be done. When you believe something can be done, really believe, your mind will find the ways to do it. Believing a solution paves the way to solution."

Porcell and I were assembling the puzzle of our dreams. We were focused on transforming ourselves and the music scene. We had a desire to create a musical culture based on a trust in the universe that everything was meant to be. A vision to see the good in whatever fate brought us. We were into healthy living and healthy mindsets. We were living in a creative city, but it had a bleak, degraded, and chaotic outlook on the world. What we were espousing was anathema to everything that was happening on the streets. We were creating an alternative, showing that it wasn't cool to be destructive and that there was a better way.

When I first arrived in the city, I was shocked to find that our record was getting attention and inspiring bands to rally behind our message. New York City was the last place I thought the straight-edge lifestyle would grow roots. But I met Raybeez, the singer of the local band Warzone, my first week in the city. He told me that *Can't Close My Eyes* had helped him and his guitarist, Todd Youth, decide to get clean from drugs and alcohol. Raybeez, a colorful comic-book character—simultaneously hero and some villain—was both feared and loved. He identified as a skinhead and wore a chain around his waist as a belt—with a lock as a belt buckle. I had known Todd since he was twelve. He was a runaway, recently released from reform school. Both Todd and Raybeez decided to get vocal about their newfound lifestyle. This was huge, because Raybeez was highly influential.

It was becoming obvious that our desire to change the world had to start with changing ourselves. We didn't complain about what society or the government was doing wrong. We focused on what we, as individuals, could do *right*. We used our music to speak our hearts on the Lower East Side, which wasn't used to hearing this kind of message. We wanted to play at more venues, so Raybeez and I started promoting our own daytime shows at the Pyramid Club on Avenue A, showcasing local bands in their teens. The Pyramid Club was a drag club in the evening, and Raybeez, Todd, and a few others from the scene got jobs there. Bikers, hardcore fans, skinheads, squatters, straight edge, and no edge all mingled at the Pyramid, proving that you could coexist peacefully while maintaining completely different ideologies.

This birthed our Saturday hardcore matinees. They had a great vibe and were a great way to showcase up-and-coming bands and attract more youth from the suburbs, who headed to the Lower East Side every weekend.

These kids had a different look from the older hardcore scene, which was dark and dirty. They were clean-cut and sober, with big black X's on both hands, which signified that they chose not to drink or smoke. The X's came from bouncers who marked the hands of underage clubgoers so they wouldn't be served alcohol but could still watch the bands. The straight-edge followers proudly displayed their desire *not* to drink, even if they were of age.

*　*　*

I got another call from 7 Seconds, who invited us to play with them throughout the Northeast and Canada. This was incredible, and it started right at the same time as Porcell's next semester at Oswego.

I called him to see if he was dropping out of college like I had done, and he assured me he was. It was summer, and he'd been staying at the apartment some nights and working a horrible landscaping job. He was saving his money to buy a new Marshall amplifier and a Gibson Les Paul guitar. Craig and Tommy, although young, were dedicated to being in a band and up for touring. Before that tour began, I booked some extra shows for us, extending down to Virginia Beach; Raleigh, North Carolina; and Washington, D.C., at the legendary 9:30 Club.

As the beginning of the tour drew near, Porcell still hadn't told his dad that he wasn't going back to school. I asked him about it every time I called him, and it was never the right time. Two days before the tour (and the start of classes), I hadn't heard from Porcell. I called in a bit of a panic. He told me not to worry and that he'd never bail.

"I'm going to tell my dad tonight," he said. "He thinks all the money I've been saving is going to college. He's so proud of me. He's going to be furious when I tell him I spent it all to buy gear."

He called me again later that night.

"What happened?" I asked. He told me about how he'd approached his dad while he was reading the newspaper and laid it out straight: He'd spent his money, was quitting school to go on tour, and planned to live with me full-time in New York. "Oh my God, how did he take it? Did he scream?"

"Worse. He was practically nonreactive," said Porcell. "He nodded, picked up his newspaper, and said, 'You're going on tour with that drifter, Cappo?'"

"He called me a *drifter*?"

"Yeah. Then he said something that really hurt," Porcell continued. "He goes, 'I really thought you were the one to make something out of your life, but it turns out that you're just going to be a loser like your loser friend, Cappo.'"

"Oh my God, that's devastating! How did you take it?"

"Whatever! It'll all work out!" He laughed to himself. "Let's go on tour."

I appreciated the simple joy and trust Porcell had. We shared a deep, inherent feeling of pronoia—a trust that the entire universe works in your favor if you are doing something good for the universe. Without ever articulating it, that was our religion. I connected the universe to a concept of God. Porcell felt it to be more like energy, but either way, we felt like we were duty bound, and we saw our work as sacred.

* * *

As the post-punk hardcore/straight-edge scene took off in New York, I developed a large circle of friends and musicians from all over the city, the country, and eventually, the world. We would hang out together on the weekends, walking the streets of the Lower East Side, going to record stores and performances, skateboarding, graffitiing, and just hanging out. I wanted to capture this time in sonic history, so my friend Jordan Cooper and I decided to create a label: Revelation Records. Many bands would come and go, and I wanted to document them before they broke up. I felt like a historian who was creating sonic archives or time capsules for future generations.

The first release was Raybeez's band Warzone. Although he called himself a skinhead, the crew he ran with was much different from the skinheads who had a political agenda or the white supremacists the media portrayed. He used the term *skinhead* as an aesthetic marker—to signal a type of fashion and musical preference, not a political leaning. He wore sleeveless flannels, calf-high Doc Martens, and superfluous suspenders. Although we were buddies and he was still clean, I was always cautious around him because of his drug history.

In addition to Todd Youth on guitar, Warzone included another young runaway named Batmite. He was from a good family in Brooklyn and looked like he was ten years old, but he was probably thirteen or fourteen. We put the record together in the simplest way possible. We could fit three and a half minutes on each side of the 7-inch record. We figured about seven Warzone songs would fit, since they were short. I contracted with a pressing plant that I discovered when I visited California, and we did the sleeve design ourselves. We also came up with the record company's logo. Since these were the days before PCs and word processors, we went to art stores and played around with rub-on letters and shapes.

I'm forever grateful that the punk/hardcore music scene taught me to be proactive. If we wanted something done—like putting out records for our friends and ourselves, booking a tour, or recording—we didn't wait around for a manager or a label. We just did it, learning from our successes and mistakes as we went. I called it the ready, fire, aim approach. Most people get stuck in preparation—ready, aim . . . and they never fire.

With Warzone, we knew we'd sell about five thousand records. The first pressing sold quickly because we packaged the records with stickers, posters, and more, like treasure chests. Soon, overseas distributors wanted to pick up the record as well, and we quickly repressed it.

One thing led to another, and we were suddenly signing bands like Gorilla Biscuits and Side by Side, both of whom opened for us at local shows. Next, we made a compilation of New York City bands, which was originally a seven-inch record but became a full-blown LP. My favorite discovery was the Sick of It All demo. They were from Queens, and I loved them. At the time, we had no idea that they and other bands would sell hundreds of thousands of records internationally.

I was naive the entire time I was doing business. I never had a business lens. I was just able to see a demand and an opportunity to preserve a moment in music history. I could see what was trending and support it. I was an influencer before that was even a thing. But I didn't capitalize on this talent. To me, the records we produced were all history, art projects, and the living experience.

* * *

Porcell had spent his last dime on his new guitar and amp. I had saved $750, so I used it to buy a 1974 cargo van. It was awesome. Not by any mechanical or aesthetic standards, but it represented a newfound freedom out of my tiny universe. To fulfill a wanderlust that was burning inside of me, and to spread Youth of Today's mission and message.

Before our dates with 7 Seconds, we set out for Virginia Beach, one of the few places I'd visited as a kid. I'd spent four summers with relatives in that seaside town, and driving there brought back the feeling of freedom and adventure that I'd experienced as a child, sitting backward in the back of the family station wagon. Ten years later, at age nineteen, I was driving my bandmates—Porcell (eighteen), Craig (fifteen), Tommy (sixteen)—and two roadies, Mark Goober (seventeen) and Matt Warnke (thirteen), the singer of Crippled Youth.

These kids all went to Porcell's high school in Katonah, New York. We got permission from the parents of the underage kids, which seems strange now. It was a cargo van, so it had no windows or seats. We had room for gear, threw a small mattress on the floor, packed light, and hit the road. We had no credit cards, no cell phones, no internet, no plan for where we would stay or what we would eat. We had two days to get to Virginia Beach. It was a complete surrender to God or the universe, trusting we'd be taken care of.

We drove all day on 95 south. When we got to Norfolk, Virginia, we pulled over and got watermelon at a roadside stand. We sat by a cornfield, and I reflected on my childhood trips to Virginia Beach. As this point, the ocean seemed like the goal. We figured we could get there by 1:30 p.m. and have the day to chill in the surf, cruise the boardwalk, and eat fudge like I had as a kid. When we started driving again, I noticed the van wasn't moving as fast as it should be. None of us knew anything about fixing cars, but we maintained a deep faith that everything would work out.

"Let's just make it to the beach," said Porcell. "We can figure it out from there."

We were topping out at 35 mph on a 55 mph road, and worry crept in. I was desperately praying, even though I didn't know whom to pray to. I had the Hail Mary memorized because our family use to say it after dinner during Lent. I was the oldest in the band and felt responsible. But we made it, rolling into the beach at sunset going 20 mph. We parked illegally and ran into the ocean. In need of a cleanse, we dove into the waves and washed away our worry and fear.

We decided to walk down Atlantic Avenue, the main drag, filled with beach food and the tourist shops that I'd loved as a child. Within fifteen minutes, we ran into two hardcore kids named Russell and Dave. They had a surfer look, wearing sun-bleached mohawks and oversized cutoff T-shirts while smoking cigarettes. We introduced ourselves, told them about the show, and asked if they knew of a place we could crash or anyone who could fix the van.

They were both mechanics of sorts and said that we could stay at their apartment, the Skull House. They were already planning to go to the show.

We couldn't have planned it better.

The Skull House was a teenage punk rock apartment that looked exactly like it sounded: garbage bags filled with beer and soda cans, dirty bathrooms, band posters and flyers stuck to the walls, random people hanging out, somebody asleep on the couch. We were grateful to have it and felt welcome and safe.

Russell and Dave had big hearts and worked on our van first thing in the morning for the entire day. It needed more time to fix, so Russell volunteered to drive us to our next show in Raleigh and back in the Skull Car, a beat-up, spray-painted sedan. Dave stayed and worked on the van. When we returned, the van *still* wasn't ready, so Dave insisted that we go north to Washington, D.C., play the 9:30 Club, then come back south again to pick up the van and head to Trenton, New Jersey, to meet up with 7 Seconds. The day we left for New Jersey, we looked at Russell and Dave like they were our saviors, heaven-sent.

We exchanged hugs and thanks and hit the road. After about thirty miles, our van started shaking violently.

"I spent $750 for this thing!" I screamed. "What a waste of good money!"

The shaking got worse and worse, and smoke started rising from the hood.

"Something's up with this thing guys," said Matt.

Then the van stopped moving entirely, right in the middle of Route 58, six hours away from Trenton.

I found Russell's number, gave it to Porcell, and told him to call him. Off he ran to look for a pay phone, traffic zipping by us. Russell and Dave came to our rescue again in the Skull Car.

"Your van is over dudes!" they said, shaking their heads. "You cracked the engine block. It's finished." We pushed the van to the side of the road, removed its plates, stuffed ourselves into the Skull Car, and made it back to the Skull House.

"Okay, listen," I said to the band. "Does anybody have *any* money?"

Nobody did.

"We've got $350 from our Virginia Beach show after playing and selling merchandise," I said. "I'm going to find a van."

Our surf saviors and I found one listed for exactly $350, a white 1970 Dodge van, the kind with a flat front and the engine between the seats. We drove outside the city to a small town, where a round, smelly, jovial man had it parked in his driveway. It was empty in the back. It had windows, but no locks on the doors. It seemed to run. We had to miss our show in Trenton, but my hope was to make the next one in Boston at the famous Rathskeller in Kenmore Square. That show would likely be sold out.

We bought it, and he gave us the title. By that point, it was 9 p.m., and we were all exhausted. Russell and Dave offered to stay up all night to make the van roadworthy, and Russell said he'd come along as a roadie, since we knew nothing about fixing vehicles. They encouraged me to go to sleep so I could wake up early and drive.

Once again, everything had worked out perfectly. We'd had just enough money to buy the new van. And we were also up one qualified roadie who was big, could carry stuff, and knew how to fix engines, flat tires, and other things we'd never learned to do. More evidence for me and Porcell that if we kept our intentions clean, the universe would work out in our favor. When we woke up at 5 a.m., Russell and Dave were just finishing work on the van.

"It's ready to go!" Dave said. "I even drilled in sliding bolts on the doors, since the locking mechanism was totally shot. You gotta lock it from the inside, then lock all the other doors and exit from the driver's door. That lock is working, at least. It's a little tricky, but it's secure now."

They even packed the van with our gear and gave us some chips and drinks. We got in, said our goodbyes to Dave, and headed off to the freeway as the morning sun was rising behind us over the Atlantic Ocean.

None of these vans had power steering, and this particular one had play in the steering wheel. I had to rock it ever so slightly to keep the van straight. It was a delicate balance, but I thought I'd gotten the hang of it by the time we got on the highway. I was wrong. The van kept swerving left and right, like I was drunk, and I couldn't seem to settle it down again. After four minutes of swerving, a state trooper pulled me over.

A well-built officer with a wide-brimmed hat came to the window, looking like an army sergeant. "License, registration, and insurance."

"Yes, officer." I reached into the glove compartment. I handed him the registration for the old van that had broken down. I'd never registered this one, just switched the plates.

"What's going on in here? Have you guys been drinking? You're swerving all over the road."

"No, sir, we're straight edge," I said. "We don't drink or smoke or take any drugs."

The officer poked his head into the van. "Who you got in this van, anyway?" The band, including thirteen-year-old Matt, were all lying down, half asleep.

"Everybody out of the van!" he shouted. "You've got no damn seats in this vehicle!"

"No, sir, we have no rear seats," I said. "It didn't come with seats in it."

We did as he said. Everyone was exhausted from the night before. Everyone except me. I was wide awake. After all, I was the oldest. I was the driver. I was the one who had the fake registration and the fake plates, and the insurance (for the other van) was in my name.

"You boys stay here. I'm going to run these plates." The officer walked back to his patrol car with its flashing lights.

I was certain that as soon as he ran the plates, I'd be caught. He'd know it was an unregistered, uninsured vehicle. What would I say then? I prayed for an appropriate response.

He walked back to our vehicle, double-checked the plates, and approached us again. He looked me square in the eyes. I looked back at him. All I wanted to do was continue the tour. I decided to do something that I'd been quite good at most of my life—play *totally* dumb.

"I'm going to ask you one time and one time only," he said. "Who's van is this?"

"It's my van." I said.

"This isn't your van, son." He spoke slowly. "These plates are registered to a 1974 Dodge. This is a 1970 Dodge. Whose van is this?"

"It's mine!" I said. "We just bought it yesterday. Here's the title. Our old 1974 Dodge van blew up yesterday. We bought this new one."

"And the plates . . . ?" He trailed off, looking confused.

"Yeah, I switched 'em. Just switched 'em over until we get home to New York," I said, as if it was no big deal.

"What do you mean," he said, getting close to my face, "you 'just switched them'?"

"I just switched 'em. Took them off the old one and just screwed them on the new one. It wasn't a big deal."

"Switched them? You can't just switch them! Are you crazy? You can't just switch plates."

"Why not? It's still registered. Don't we get some type of grace period?"

"No! You have to wait until the DMV opens on Monday morning and bring it to get registered."

"We can't wait until Monday," I said, still playing dumb. "Matt's got to get home to his parents." I gestured to Matt, who was looking slightly helpless with his sleepy morning face and wrinkled, dirty clothes. "His mom wants him back."

"Are you out of your mind, kid?" the officer said. "I could have you all arrested and this van impounded. You've got no seat belts. You've got no *seats*! Your van is unregistered and uninsured!"

"Officer, we have good intentions," I said, throwing myself on his mercy. "We're not out doing drugs or driving drunk. We're just a bunch of kids traveling around, seeing this country, and making music. We need to get up north *today*. We can't wait till Monday. I'm sorry. Please let us go."

He heard what I said, digested it, and inhaled deeply. Time stood still.

"Okay." He nodded. A glimmer of hope. "Get out of here. "Get in your van and get out of this state."

We thanked him profusely. Everyone jumped in the back, quickly falling back to sleep. Only Porcell, Russell, and I stayed awake. I tried to skillfully steer the van so it went straight, which required incredible diligence.

Porcell sat shotgun. "It always works out for the best," he said with a smile.

We drove west and then north as the heat started to bake us in that four-wheeled tin box with no air conditioning. The engine cooked us up well in that early September humidity.

Tommy, our drummer, suddenly quit while we were driving and asked us to take him back to New York City on the way to Boston. After a flurry of calls at a pay phone, we secured another drummer, Drew Thomas, who finished that tour with us. He was fourteen years old.

That $350 unregistered, uninsured Dodge van took us to Boston, Albany, Syracuse (although we missed the show because I got lost), Toronto, Chicago, Detroit, and back to New York City. As the opener for 7 Seconds, we played packed shows and met new fans who ended up becoming loyal followers. Most of all, we learned a lesson in trust.

After three months of taking us around NYC, that van finally died on Fourteenth Street. We took off the plates and left it for dead between Seventh and Eighth Avenues, headed east. I never did get around to registering it.

*   *   *

After the tour, Porcell, his friend Gavin—who'd recently moved to the city—and I got late-night barback jobs at the Tunnel, an 80,000-square-foot railroad terminal turned disco on Twelfth Avenue. Even though none of us did drugs, drank, or danced, the energy and the money were enticing. The Tunnel was the Studio 54 of the 1980s. One of the dance floors had abandoned railroad tracks that went off into a tunnel, into the darkness. It was a *very* cool concept. The club was massive, with multiple rooms on multiple levels. It was packed every night, kicking off the party at about 11 p.m. Our jobs introduced us to a new scene of young people who were more artistic or more into New York nightlife than the hardcore and straight-edge crowds.

In the 1980s, all the alternative scenes were more or less a melting pot. I got a cool club girlfriend, too. She wasn't straight edge at all, but she was fun and had a good attitude. Porcell, Gavin, and I walked around dressed in black, the music and energy pulsing through our veins as we collected empty beer bottles and glasses in busboy tubs and hauled them to the dishwashing station. Occasionally, we helped bartenders cut up lemons and limes and haul cases of beer. But that was it, the whole job. And the money was decent because of the tips.

There was a sense of giddiness and expectation, layered with a tangible feeling of sexual opportunity—a fun atmosphere for a twenty-year-old. Plus, it was *our* hangout. We were on the inside. It was a frenetic party atmosphere, with gorgeous people, celebrities, and cocaine. On any given night, you might see Mike Tyson, RuPaul, Jam Master Jay, Lady Bunny, or Arnold Schwarzenegger. Vin Diesel worked security. All kinds of sex happened in the bathrooms. We witnessed all of the excitement, but didn't indulge in any of it.

And then, all of a sudden, it just wasn't fun anymore. The party got old and sad pretty quickly. The club scene was full of people using fame or beauty as currency. It started to remind me of high school. I realized just how shallow it was and that it brought out the shallowness within me.

I had moved to New York City to escape a vapid existence based on external gratification. I understood that people wanted to get together and become vulnerable and intimate. I understood the importance of community and that alcohol could make a shy person reveal their true self. But I wasn't looking for that. I had written down a quote from one of the yoga books I was reading: "Pleasure for the ego will manifest in pain." I felt that pain at the Tunnel. The more I dove into my spiritual study, the more I realized that the nightclub scene did not align with what I wanted to become. The excitement left me feeling gross. Defiled, as the Buddha says.

One day, I read the *Dhammapada* 13.167, and it hit me hard, like a plank to the temple: "Follow not the vulgar way, live not in heedlessness, hold not false views, linger not long in worldly existence."

This was my telegram from God. What I needed to pull the plug. I was lingering in worldly existence. I wanted a better way. I needed to quit my job and move on.

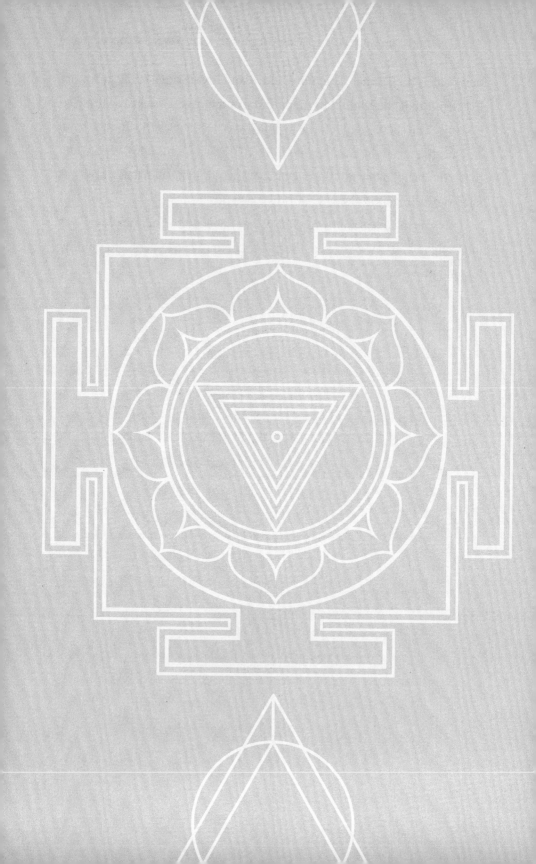

CHAPTER 4

THE KRISHNAS & BHAKTI YOGA

I loved underground hardcore music. It had grown out of the punk rock of the late 1970s, getting faster and louder, with more screaming than singing. Songs were powerful and short, sometimes a minute and a half or less. There were very few records of the bands that were playing. Antidote, a band I loved, did have a record: eight songs of buzz-saw guitar and screeching vocals that could work anyone into a frenzy. The picture on the record sleeve depicted a man about to swing an axe at the head of a pitiful cow, except their heads were swapped. The man had an angry cow's head, and the cow had a desperate human face. The title of the EP was *Thou Shalt Not Kill.*

One day, while walking down Eighth Street, I saw a white lady dressed in a sari. She was standing by a book table with a strange statue—a man with the head of a cow about to slaughter a cow with the head of a man.

"Wow, it's the Antidote cover come to life!" I joked to Porcell.

The lady, who I thought would be oblivious to my quip, said, "Antidote? Yes, I know Louie and Nunzio." They were the singer and guitarist.

How did this Krishna devotee know Antidote, an obscure and awesome hardcore band? She handed me a card to her apartment on Greenwich Avenue, where on Mondays, Tuesdays, and Thursdays she held yoga classes. The card read: "Bhakti Yoga Classes, Mantra Meditation, Bhagavad Gita Study & Free Vegetarian Feast." I was intrigued. It was two blocks from my apartment. "Please, come to kirtan. It's spiritual singing and call-and-response chanting."

I nodded, but I didn't know what she was talking about.

"Sometimes Louie comes," she said. "Do you know Cro-Mags?"

My jaw dropped. "Wait. You know Cro-Mags?"

"Yes," she said. "Harley was just here helping us distribute food in the park to the homeless."

Two days later, my friend Richie convinced me to go to the Greenwich Avenue class and kirtan. I was excited and a little hesitant because the Krishnas seemed to have a cultlike vibe. When I arrived at the front door, I could smell the delicious aroma of Indian spices. We were buzzed in. We made our way to the second floor, and sure enough, a bunch of scenesters from the hardcore community were there, seemingly out of place in the sacred room. It was a nice, big-windowed space with sparse furniture and oak floors. There was an altar with small statues. It was decorated with flowers, an incense holder, and small framed pictures of the late guru and founder of the Krishna Consciousness movement, A. C. Bhaktivedanta Swami, and other Indian gods and goddesses. I saw a bookshelf filled with sacred literature.

Some people around my age were dressed as monks, wearing kurtas, or tunics. I didn't recognize them, but they had a few tattoos, which led me to think they were hardcore kids that had been zapped and converted. There were more white women in saris and an older man with a beautiful smile who seemed as though he was going to lead the group.

The smell of the incense and spices was overpowering. The droning sound of the chanting kicked in as people sat down. I was slightly weirded out, but there were enough outsiders and hardcore scenesters there to make me feel at ease. One lady, dressed normally, chanted with a beautiful smile on her face as if she was either in complete ecstasy or fully indoctrinated by the cult. I wasn't quite sure which it was. But her happiness was inspiring. I wondered how chanting could make a person so blissful . . . and why I was upset by another person's bliss.

Although I was starting to feel attacked, I was excited for the free Indian food, which was vegetarian, and I wanted to learn the *Bhagavad Gita*, which is considered a classic book of wisdom in the yoga tradition. I wasn't sure what they meant about a free bhakti yoga class, because I didn't see anywhere to do yoga. Then I learned that bhakti yoga wasn't necessarily a physical practice like an asana class. It was a spiritual practice.

We sat on cushions. The singer was chanting on a harmonium, an instrument with a Western pianolike keyboard, reeds, and an accordionlike pump. Harmoniums are European, but they arrived in India during the mid-nineteenth century, most likely brought there by missionaries or traders. They were adopted into Indian, Pakistani, and Bangladeshi music and had become popular in the US yoga community and among kirtan enthusiasts. Somebody else played a bright-yellow clay Indian drum I'd never seen before. It had one head the size of a peanut butter jar lid and another the size of a paper plate. Chanters deftly played karatalas, hand cymbals.

Everyone looked strangely blissful, which made me even more skeptical. Were they feeling some internal joy? Why didn't I feel it? I couldn't get into it. My inner New Yorker wouldn't allow it. I looked around the room, judging everyone, including Raybeez, who sat next to me. He was about a decade older than me, putting him just shy of thirty, perhaps, which made him a punk lifer. I started wondering if that's who I wanted to be. Would I ever want to grow up and have a conventional life? Or would I eschew material life forever like Raybeez? He was covered in poorly done tattoos, a public declaration in those days that said, "Don't hire me. I'm going to live in this world as an outcast. And I'm okay with that."

After the chanting, the leader spoke some mantras in Sanskrit (which he then translated for us), starting with verse 2.13 of the *Bhagavad Gita*:

> As the embodied soul continuously passes in this
> life from childhood, to youth, to old age, the soul
> similarly enters a new body at the time of death.
> Those who are wise are not bewildered by such
> a change.

He put down the book and smiled, lighting up the room. "We are souls that have a body," he said. "We are not white or Black or Asian or American or European. We are not male or female. These are the designations of the body. We fight, oppress, try to lord over others due to a particular body type. But according to the *Gita*, we are all very similar. Spiritual beings driving in a vehicle made up of matter. To quote C. S. Lewis, 'We do not have a soul; we are a soul that has a material body.' This is what the *Gita* teaches."

My skepticism began to take a back seat. What he was saying resonated with me. He explained that the body will always change and that the spirit will witness this change. Only out of ignorance does one think the body is the same as the self. He spoke about the equal rights and equality that we wanted, but asked us to consider where that equality lies. He told us how we tended to draw a circle around white males and that we needed to make that circle wider. It wasn't enough to draw it over white men and women, either. We needed to draw that circle around all nations. All nationalities. All pigments of skin.

But then he asked us if that was where commonality stopped. He asked us why animals were judged differently simply because they had different bodies. This was what I had been trying to explain to my family on Thanksgiving, after I'd become vegetarian.

The speaker explained that we couldn't fix the problems of inequality on the material level—there was no equality on a material level. We had to take it to the spiritual level because our bodies and minds would never be equal. Equality had to be found in a more subtle way, what great yogis of the past described as the equality of the soul. Further, when we thought of the body as our self, we would spend our life trying to fulfill the needs of the body, which was futile. The desires of the body were insatiable, according to Buddhists.

"The senses always want more," he said, paraphrasing the Buddha. "This is what addiction is. You're feeding the body. It's making you sick, addicted, broke, or destitute, and yet you still want more. The desires are never-ending. The cup is never filled. Fulfilling desires of the mind and body only *increases* one's desires. Has anyone else experienced that? I know I have."

I thought again about Raybeez, before he got clean, and the other addicts within the punk scene. Even the people who only came to the Lower East Side to score dope. They used to be citizens wearing suits, but they became disheveled zombies, strung out on the street as if somebody had kidnapped their souls. It made me sad to see them falling asleep as they tried to beg for change. They fed themselves the drug, but it never sated them. And in the meantime, many had lost everything they held dear—families, careers, marriages, savings.

"The *soul* is what needs to be fed," the speaker said. "There's no amount of alcohol, heroin, cocaine, pizza, or corn chips that can satisfy the soul. We live in a culture of overconsumption"—he paused here for effect—"and our souls are starved." He let the statement sink in for a moment, then asked, "Does anyone think their soul is hungry?"

I observed his joyful face, enraptured.

"We're going to honor prasad," he said, referencing sacred food. "We don't eat prasad. We honor it. Because it's offered to Lord Vishnu, it's nondifferent from Vishnu."

I didn't quite understand what he meant by this and was afraid that we weren't going to eat after all. I'd been here for an hour and a half, and I was hungry. But then some younger monks brought out buckets filled with Indian food and lined them up to be served. We chanted a little longer, then dug in.

I saw Louie eating with some other skinheads and mohawk kids from the scene. They sat in a circle, wearing all of their punk rock armor except for their boots. At that point, my band and I no longer dressed outlandishly. We'd traded in the punk look for the clean-cut skater look: shaved heads or bleached-blond hair, high-tops or Vans with board shorts, Champion sweatshirts, and tight jeans rolled up high. It was cutting edge at the time, even though it's normal today.

Harley rolled in just in time for the food. He sat down next to me. I never knew what to say to him, since I both feared and worshiped him.

"Perfect timing," I said, making obvious small talk. "Skip all that chanting stuff and arrive for the food!"

He scoffed. "No, man, I love the chanting and the *Bhagavad Gita*. I was just late 'cause I had practice."

I felt stupid. *One of these days, he's going to kick my ass.*

The food was good. Turmeric rice with raisins, vegetable curry, moong dal, and cardamom halva. It wasn't just good food. There was something special about it. I'd been to vegetarian restaurants, but this was different. I smiled as I was eating it.

A young monk with tattoos came over to me. "Do you like the prasad? This is food made with love."

"What do you mean?"

"It's prepared with love. That's why it's different," he said. "We're not making it for profit like some guy with unclean habits who owns a restaurant. Those unclean habits get transferred into the food you're eating. If the guy is lustful or angry or a criminal, you're eating that bullshit." He was clearly a hardcore guy turned monk. I loved that he used the words *bullshit* and *unclean habits* in the same breath, parroting the language of books that weren't part of his vernacular. I recognized him as a bike messenger who rode a single gear around the Lower East Side. He had a forearm of black-ink tattoos, but he looked saintly in his saffron robe and kurta. "It's not just vegetarian food, it's prasad. You're eating the love and devotion of the cook."

Now, decades later, I know that it's common in holy cities throughout India for someone to walk up to you and hand you prasad, a sacred offering of food. It's a gesture of love. Food is cooked in loving meditation to the deity. It's offered with love and then distributed to the community. The idea is that prasad is karma-free and awakens the soul. After all, the main ingredient is love, something our prepackaged and frozen foods are significantly deficient in.

I don't know how India got pigeonholed as the country with starving people. For more than thirty-five years, I've been invited to so many sacred feasts and handed free offerings of prasad so many times that it's almost expected now. The distribution of prasad is not limited to the homeless or the poor. The idea is that we are all starving. We're just starving for love, and therefore it's given to any who will accept it.

I began going there regularly to eat this food cooked with love.

*　　*　　*

I started dating Stacia, a girl who practiced Buddhism. She was fit, sexy, smart, and spiritually minded. She went to Columbia University and knew about my interest in all things spiritual. By this point, I was a big fan of Buddhist literature, particularly the Tipitaka (or Pali canon), a collection texts that form the doctrinal foundation of Theravada Buddhism. My favorite was the *Dhammapada*, the book I'd brought to Bible study and perhaps the most widely read Buddhist text. Most Buddhists don't worship a personal God, although the Mahayana tradition takes the form of devotion to the Buddha himself and the bodhisattvas, or enlightened masters. Sometimes the devoted will sit on the floor facing the deity of the Buddha and chant mantras. I found the teachings beautiful, universal, and timeless: *Desire causes pain. There are good and bad thoughts. Good and bad deeds. Good and bad speech. Respect life. Keep the mind clean. Uproot suffering.* I was excited when she invited me to a local Buddhist gathering.

There were about eighteen students gathered in a circle on the floor in one of the campus buildings. The room was dimly lit, and the impressive architecture of Columbia University added charm to the experience. Frankincense burned on the bookshelf. The group leader read some passages from a book that seemed steeped in wisdom. The other students were my age and casually dressed. I introduced myself, and after a few niceties and introductions, the leader started speaking.

"We're going to start chanting. Repeat after me."

They led me through the mantra syllable by syllable: *Nam myoho renge kyo.* Then we sat and chanted for about ten minutes. After a while, we started sounding like the buzzing of bees, which I felt was auspicious. A transcendent hum.

After the chanting, I raised my hand. The leader of the group called on me. He wasn't a priest, per se. He was most likely a student who studied these teachings more than the others. Nobody in this group seemed ordained or anything official.

"What is the meaning of all this?" I asked. "What are we chanting for?"

"This mantra is considered to be the essence of Buddhist mantras and can grant so many benefits, including developing your Buddha-nature," he said. I had heard of Buddha-nature—a state of pure consciousness—and it was attractive. My material nature had been problematic for my entire life. Then he said something that caught me off guard. "I also use it to get what I need."

"What do you mean?" I asked.

"Well, my car broke down, and I needed a new car. I set my intention on that, continued using my mantras, and somebody offered me a car a few days later."

The students' faces lit up. Another student raised his hand. "I wanted a mountain bike, and I got one practically the next day. All from the chanting."

Confused, I raised my hand. "The entire teaching of Buddhism, and you can correct me if I'm wrong, is that 'stuff' causes more desires. Why are we chanting for more stuff?" I found myself mimicking some of the lessons I'd heard in those *Bhagavad Gita* classes on Greenwich Avenue. "Didn't the Buddha himself teach that desires cause pain? And that fulfilling desires just makes you want more? And that desires cannot be extinguished by trying to fulfill them? It's only by the absence of desire that we can obtain peace? Didn't he teach that? And shouldn't our mantras give us Buddhahood, God, or enlightenment instead of stuff? After all, we're going to lose all our stuff when we die. And breaking our attachment to all the stuff we have will cause even more pain when we have to relinquish it at the cruel hands of death." My voice kept rising in pitch. "What's the point of stuff, anyway? Cluttering up our heads, our lives. How do we squeeze lasting satisfaction from *stuff*? We're all going to die!"

I was basically pouring out everything I'd written in my journals over the last few months and unleashing it on this Buddhist group. "Why would I be praying for stuff? Mantras should bring us to the love of God."

This was met with dead silence.

Finally, one of the other teenagers spoke up. "Well, what mantra *should* we chant?"

"Well, I'm not a Krishna, but those guys down on Greenwich Avenue say that if you chant *their* mantra, you get rid of all your desires and just fall in love with God."

Later that night, I lay next to Stacia on her dorm room floor on some cushions we'd pushed together. I was disturbed. I stared at the crown molding, thinking about the Buddhist gathering. Stacia tried to get snuggly, but I knew sexual intimacy wasn't something I wanted, even though I was attracted to her. My sex drive was strong. It had dominated me for years, owning my thoughts. It had caused me to make a fool of myself and shatter hearts. I didn't want drugs or alcohol to make me act against my better judgment, and I didn't want any other desire to do so either. Sex seemed like a piece of frosted cake with shards of glass in it, a sweetness fused with emotional pain. It was never what it appeared to be or what I imagined it would be. Reality was less erotic than fantasy, yet the urge was demanding and unrelenting. My spiritual path was forcing me to distinguish between the urge and the reality.

The fact that Stacia was very attractive *and* liked me was an ego boost. I had never been the guy to attract beautiful women. But as I lay on the floor with her, I wondered about love in the material world. Was that all it was? An ego boost? A feeling of importance because my girlfriend was sexy? And her feeling important because her boyfriend sang in a band? It seemed foolish. We could enjoy sex for a few moments. We could go out together and impress a few people. Big deal.

She tried to kiss me, but I turned away and decided to tell her what I was thinking.

"I don't mean this in a bad way," I said, "because I find you very attractive. I've had sex. But it's not what I need in *this* relationship."

She looked puzzled.

"I don't know you that well," I continued, "and I don't want to go there yet. Or maybe ever."

Maybe I was a fool, potentially sabotaging all future sex with the prettiest girl I had ever dated. But I didn't understand why sex had to come into the picture. I wasn't sure if love and sex could be untangled from one another.

"I'm sorry if I made a scene at the gathering today," I said. "I didn't mean to. I'm just sick of the world of stuff. Those guys didn't seem like they embraced the teachings of the Buddha." I didn't want to use mantras like a metaphysical Sears catalog.

I continued staring at the ceiling, and eventually Stacia, with her perfectly sculpted beauty, fell asleep. I'm sure she was confused. I'm sure men didn't usually turn her down. But it wasn't about her. My soul wanted love, but my body and mind seemed to want pure lust. I tried to observe her objectively, scientifically. What was it that made me desire her? Was it her shape? Hips? Waist? What made a particular form intrinsically attractive? Was it just the way our brains worked?

I wondered if beauty made sex more enjoyable. Beauty seemed mental, and sex seemed physical. I felt that the entire act of sex, which was often mislabeled as *making love*, was an irreconcilable and incongruous desire. I thought I understood the difference between love and lust. *Love* meant I wanted to serve, respect, and hold someone or something in the highest regard. *Lust* meant I wanted to take something to fill a hole in my heart.

I had been trying to understand these forces since tenth grade, when I was obsessed with a girl in my math class. I'd called it love. I didn't even know her, but I thought I was in love with her. I leered at her every day like a cat fixated on a mouse. I loved her perfect hair. I loved her perfect legs. I loved her perfect smile. I loved her perfect breasts.

One day, I started to ask myself some questions: *Would you love her if you couldn't ever kiss her? Would you love her without any physical or sexual indulgence whatsoever? If you love her, you should be able to be with her without these things.*

I decided that I couldn't and that my version of love was hopelessly entangled with lust. I couldn't say I would still be infatuated with her if she suddenly lost a limb or gained weight. And now, lying next to Stacia, I wondered if love should only be reserved for a higher power.

After that, I would no longer say "I love you" in my mind or to anyone. I could lust after anyone instantly. But to *love* somebody? It was a different thing. Lust came from lower, darker regions. Love came from a celestial plane. Lust disregarded the person, making her into an object. This dehumanization was the gateway to misogyny. Love couldn't be that cheap.

I decided to stop dating—at least for a while—and journal about it more.

*　*　*

I was confused about my spiritual quest. Although I connected with the teachings of the Buddha, the universe was pointing me toward Vedic culture and the *Bhagavad Gita*. Toward mantras. Toward kirtan. Toward meditation. Toward exclusive devotion. Yet the only people I knew who were into bhakti yoga, or at least who took it seriously and didn't just attend classes for the free food, were Harley Flanagan and his followers—a lawless, violent, pot-smoking street gang.

One day, Porcell and I were locking up our bikes in front of a health-food store when Harley Flanagan and his friends came out—a mix of camouflage fatigues, black-ink tattoos, and sacred tulasi beads. Their moustaches were green from drinking wheatgrass. They were an intimidating bunch.

"We're fired up," said Harley. "We're going to CBGB, and we're going to kick Billy Psycho's ass."

Billy Psycho, the drummer for the Psychos, was twice Harley's size. Sure, it would be an intriguing brawl, but where did this violence fit in to his spiritual calling? Harley was the first person to encourage me to read the *Bhagavad Gita*. Why was he always kicking people's asses when he and his crew had stopped wearing leather shoes, citing animal cruelty? Similarly, I loved Cro-Mags's fiery, powerful music, but it brought out my anger. I was afraid it was tearing me away from a spiritual calling. I was trying to figure out who I was, and these mixed signals didn't help.

Were all the Krishnas part of a cult, where you could act as crazy as you wanted? They said bhakti yoga was the yoga of love, but the *Bhagavad Gita* took place on a battlefield. My heart was burning for clarity. Later, I realized that some people might get inspired by a spiritual quest, but that didn't necessarily mean they represented the highest standard of the path. I never stopped appreciating Harley for what he gave me.

But at that time, I knew I was devoted to God—I just didn't know who or what God was. I could recognize the commonality in spiritual teachings, but I wanted a regular practice and commitment.

Meanwhile, as I wrestled with these spiritual questions, Porcell and I found it hard to land jobs. We didn't want to compromise our ability to tour or get gigs. A regular job would have done just that. But we had an idea. We drew up a flyer that read, "College students will clean your house, paint, or do odd jobs—$10 an hour." At the bottom, we wrote our phone number twenty times so that it could be easily torn off. Our business skyrocketed immediately. For us, it was great money because our rent was only $248. We'd easily make that and cover our food costs. Plus, our hours were flexible and our cash was under the table.

One morning, I got a call from a man named Joshua who asked if I could clean his office. It was right around the corner from our apartment. I walked up Seventh Avenue, took a right on the south side of the street, and located the address. A thin, well-dressed man in his late thirties or early forties marched down the stairs to greet me. He paused, squinting at the tulasi beads wrapped twice around my neck like a choker.

"Are you a devotee?" Joshua asked.

I didn't know what to say. I'd bought these beads at the Krishna temple. I understood that they meant you were devoted to God, so I supposed that in the broadest sense of the word I *was* devoted to God. That's how I answered.

"Yes, I am."

He nodded. "Please come upstairs."

I could smell incense burning and immediately saw a framed picture of the Hindu deities Radha and Krishna, the divine feminine and masculine.

Then I saw a framed picture of Chaitanya Mahaprabhu and another of A. C. Bhaktivedanta Swami.

I wondered if this was another Krishna temple. Was Krishna mystically following me? I understood recency bias, the theory that something you've just learned about seems to appear everywhere. But this was getting too weird. Aside from the framed pictures, Joshua gave no outward indication that he was a Krishna devotee.

"Where *am* I?" I asked.

"This is Bala Books," he said. "We publish children's books on Krishna Consciousness."

"You don't look like a Krishna devotee," I said. "You look like a normal man running a business . . . with hair."

"External outfits are just that, Ray. External." He spoke with wisdom and maturity. "I've found that what really matters is what's *internal*."

I nodded. It seemed like this person had been sent to me. He was relatable and approachable, and I immediately sensed a sober truthfulness about him.

"Why don't you have a Sanskrit name?" I asked. "Your name is Joshua?"

"I do have one. I use it sometimes. It's Yogeshwara Das. Yogeshwara is a name for Krishna that means he's the master of the yogis, and Das means I am a servant of his."

"Wow. You're *actually* a Krishna devotee? The only Krishna devotees I know are gang members! What's that about?" I asked. "Are you into violence, too?"

"I don't know what you're talking about," he said.

Perhaps he'd never met any of the Cro-Mags.

"What's up with the Krishnas? Are those guys for real?"

I felt I could talk to him frankly, and he would give me a straight answer.

"Krishna is a way to say God," he said. "There's one God, but God has many names in many cultures. Religions are different ways to approach the same God. But God is one. We're here to remember what we forgot: that we're all connected and that we're all a part of something greater than us."

I nodded, accepting what he was saying.

"A. C. Bhaktivedanta Swami I can vouch for," Joshua said. "I traveled with him around Europe when I was a young man living in France. I had the fortune of serving him personally. He was a pure devotee of God. A genuine master."

*   *   *

After the odd jobs gig, I got a job in a vegetarian restaurant on First Avenue and Ninth Street called Ahimsa. I started as a dishwasher, then a short-order cook, and later a waiter. *Ahimsa* means "nonviolence" in Sanskrit. I loved working there. I loved meeting the people who came in. They were all conscious eaters, peculiar yogis, macrobiotic enthusiasts, or avant-garde scenesters. A bunch of guys from the hardcore scene worked there, too, including some that were devotees of Krishna or into yoga. I started to learn how to cook for myself at Ahimsa, and I met many people who believed in a cruelty-free diet. It propelled me to go deeper into my convictions about vegetarianism and animal rights.

The owner of Ahimsa was a devotee of Swami Satchidananda from the Integral Yoga Institute, a yoga studio and health-food store near my apartment on the West Side. He also owned a health-food store called Prana, where Porcell got a job. There was a third store called Ayurveda, a bookstore right next to Prana. Even though it was called Ayurveda, it was more of an alternative bookstore, as the ancient teaching of Indian medicine and healing wasn't very popular in the United States yet. At that time, there were probably only one or two books published on Ayurvedic medicine in the West.

Ayurveda carried books on alternative diets, alternative spirituality, fasting, the teachings of various gurus of India and Southeast Asia, mysticism, witchcraft, yoga, the occult, reincarnation, and all the other stuff that fascinated and allured me. I'd spend hours sitting on the floor, reading book after book, drinking it all up. There was one book on Ayurveda that intrigued me so much that I bought it, but I found it difficult to grasp. I knew there was wisdom there, but I needed a teacher. I also genuinely wanted to figure out how to thrive on a vegetarian diet, since I found myself exhausted and lethargic. I suspected I wasn't getting as much protein as I needed. I ate healthy food. I got it for free or discounted from the restaurant and Prana. I was physically active—always biking, walking, or running—but I was tired all the time. I also had chronic indigestion and acid reflux, something I'd struggled with since age sixteen. I was addicted to taking over-the-counter antacid tablets.

One day while reading, I saw the shop owner giving what seemed to be medical advice for herbs, supplements, and tinctures to a customer. As I eavesdropped, I noticed it was Ayurvedic advice, and I stopped what I was reading and rushed to the counter.

"Are you an Ayurvedic doctor?" I asked. "I just bought this book on Ayurveda and I can't figure it out."

"Yes," he said. "My name is Bhagavat."

Bhagavat had long red hair, a beard, and a carefully combed mustache. He was tall, thin, and healthy looking. He told me to come back the next day at 2 p.m. I brought a list of questions for him, and I told him about my fatigue and indigestion.

"You cannot diagnose someone by merely hearing of a symptom," said Bhagavat. "Everybody has a unique physical constitution and will require a unique remedy. Ayurveda takes the entire constitution of the client's body and lifestyle into consideration. It also considers the seasons, the weather, their age, what time they go to bed, what they do for a living—all these things influence our well-being. We are *signature* beings, Ray, and therefore we need a signature health protocol that fits who we are."

I thought this was brilliant.

He felt my pulse and had me open my eyes wide.

"Do you eat on top of undigested food?"

"What do you mean?"

"Do you eat, and then before you digest your food, do you eat again? Like twenty minutes later? Or an hour later?"

"I work at Ahimsa, right up the block. I eat all day. All day!" I said. "But everything I eat is organic and vegetarian. It's *very* healthy. I get all my food from the health-food store. I even drink a sixteen-ounce glass of spirulina and water every day!" I felt a bit defensive.

"It doesn't matter if it's healthy or not," Bhagavat said. "Your digestion can only take so much food. The yogis envision digestion as a fire, or jatharagni, a heat in the body. Imagine I'm holding up a flaming matchstick, and you put five big logs on top of it. It would go out immediately. But if you put that same match on tinder such as newspapers and straw and gradually increase the size of the wood and sticks and *then* add logs, you'll have a bonfire."

He explained that if I was snacking all day, I was not eating healthy, even if the food itself was wholesome. I was packing my digestive system with more food than it could handle. He told me that because my body was kind, it was sending extra acid to help me break down the extra food.

"That acid is a gift from God," he said. "And how are you repaying that gift? You're taking these pills to neutralize the acid."

He looked at me kindly, shaking his head. He warned me that if I didn't let my body digest what I'd already consumed, I could develop other symptoms. He recommended that I fast until noon the next day and sip plenty of hot water. I was also to stop eating at 6:30 p.m., or four hours before I went to bed, for one week.

"Do this every day this week and come back and tell me how you're feeling," he said.

I hadn't been expecting this advice, but it made sense. I loved a big breakfast, and I was always exhausted after I ate it. He also told me not to drink water or other liquid right before meals, during meals, or right after meals.

"Just sip that hot water all morning and flush your system," he said. "Then, stop an hour before your lunch and you'll be ready to eat. This should be an easy fix if you take it seriously." I nodded obediently, but I was resistant. I loved snacking, and I loved the food at the restaurant. "Ray, we live in a world where everybody wants a pill to make things change. There's no quick fix. In Ayurveda, we're trying to correct our lifestyle so we don't have these emergencies. You're young. You can do this. You have a responsibility to this body. It's a gift, and therefore you should maintain it and take care of it."

"Are you sure it's just not an acid problem?"

"Ray," he said, "hear me. Stopping the symptom of the problem will not stop the problem. You can poke out the fuel light on your dashboard, but if you ignore it, you'll have a bigger problem."

In the end, I followed Bhagavat's advice. And I never had acid reflux again.

*　　*　　*

A lot of the people who came to Ahimsa were incredibly interesting. At that time, most people who cared enough about vegetarian food to seek out a restaurant were alternative thinkers, bohemians on the fringe of society. This was great for me as someone who loved talking and meeting people when business was slow.

Jennifer, a restaurant regular, was an asset on my spiritual journey. She studied yoga, and I told her that I was looking for a qualified teacher. She highly recommended hers, Dharma Mittra, who taught out of his studio in the West Village. While I wasn't interested in mastering backbends and handstands, I felt yogic wisdom was an inclusive understanding of spirituality, and I needed some spiritual grounding and instruction. I yearned to learn the yogic truths.

In the 1980s, yoga in the United States focused on spirituality, and every center leaned toward a classical practice, such as mantra, pranayama, and asana. There wasn't a secularized yoga studio on every corner like there is today. The teachers had depth and poise. They were learned.

Jennifer told me to meet her at the studio. The entrance was in an alley between two buildings. In the window there was a tacky neon sign that read "OM" and "Dharma Mittra Yoga." The floor was carpeted, and incense burned, wafting spirals of scented smoke. Pictures of former teachers from throughout the years were delicately placed in a row next to each other. Those people looked as if they were from another time, if not another planet. They wore big beads around their necks and clay markings on their foreheads. They were either bare-chested or in robes. The women, wrapped in saris, looked angelic, with softened features and bindi on their foreheads.

The gurus were either jovial or grave in the photographs. Most were laughing or appeared to be thinking deeply on lofty topics that were probably out of my grasp. Framed posters of Ganesh and Shiva, with whom I was barely acquainted, gave a feeling of otherworldliness. I also spotted a framed poster of Kali, wearing a garland of skulls and holding a trident and sword, and another of Gene Simmons with his tongue sticking out of his mouth.

There was an altar with brass statues of Hindu deities, pictures of Indian masters, and incense. Even though I didn't understand much about any of it, the masters seemed sacred, and the place felt like hallowed ground. On a nearby bookshelf, I noticed a copy of the *Bhagavad Gita*, alongside *Light on Yoga* by B. K. S. Iyengar and books by Swami Sivananda, a Vedic spiritual teacher who passed away in 1963.

The class was small, about fifteen people, and they looked serious. I rolled out a mat next to a gaunt man with a long, thin face, sporting skin-tight bikinilike shorts. He was extremely flexible. I was not.

Dharma entered. He was a small, beautiful, soft-spoken Brazilian man. He had a charming smile and the body of a gymnast. I went up to introduce myself, and he gently bowed his head and offered the anjali mudra, or namaste greeting, hands pressed together at the chest with fingers pointed upward. I wasn't yet used to this greeting, but it was business as usual for him. Dharma was a modern-day sadhu. I told him I was new to a physical practice, but I was here to learn about all the spiritual facets of the yoga system.

In a soft yet animated voice he said, "First, we must learn to calm the tumultuous mind. There can be no peace when the mind is tumultuous. If there is no peace, how can there be happiness?"

I wasn't sure if I was supposed to answer, so I just nodded.

"Let's sit down and breathe and slow the mind."

Jennifer appeared and set up her mat next to mine. We did fifteen minutes of breathing techniques. Breathing, which I normally did on autopilot, was now conscious, deep, and regulated. With my right thumb I sealed my right nostril and then began slowly and precisely inhaling through the left. At the top of my breath I sealed the left nostril and released my right for a long, controlled exhale. At the bottom of the breath, I inhaled through the right again. The entire time, my middle finger was tapping my third eye.

"This alternate-nostril breathing will bring peace to your mind, balance to your nervous system, and lower blood pressure," Dharma said softly but loud enough for us to hear. His voice, soothing and confident, was enough to lower my blood pressure. I felt peaceful. Stress and anxiety started to melt. I noticed that my mind, usually racing all over the place, was now relaxed and settled. I knew this simple, regulated breathing was good for me. It was sort of like a trance. It got me out of my planning or looking-toward-the-future mode. I was in being-here mode, which was completely foreign to me.

The physical class was a workout, and my sweatpants and sweatshirt were *not* needed. I should have worn bikini briefs like the guy next to me. Even though I considered myself athletic, I couldn't keep up with the class. I was hot and unsteady. Jennifer and the guy in bikini briefs moved gracefully, like dancers, their breathing controlled.

Dharma saw me struggling. "Why are you holding your breath?" he asked calmly. You must breathe."

Easier said than done. My default was to grip, squint, bite my lip, furrow my brow, and hold my breath. Sometimes I sighed or groaned as if I were lifting weights, though the room was otherwise church-quiet. When it was time to do headstands, I was the only one who couldn't do them. At first I couldn't understand why I was struggling. I was healthy, wasn't I?

One of my many yoga books explained that the spirit soul is trapped and struggling in this body and in the mind. I felt trapped in both. The goal of yoga is to be a jivanmukta, a person whose spirit is free or transcendental and no longer burdened by the body and mind.

I left that class, but I had some hope that yoga practice would still be a good thing for me.

* * *

At some point, I was sick of hearing myself. I used to enjoy being a big mouth. Clever. Sarcastic. Rude. Stinging. Cruel. I made people laugh. But my humor was always at another's expense. My bandmates and I bonded by insulting each other. I had a lot of practice at tearing people down, and I was vicious, targeting the way they looked or behaved. After the ego boost I got from making people laugh, I never felt very good. I felt bad for the person I humiliated, usually a close friend. I was known to lash out during road trips, idle conversations, and performances.

One day, my phone rang as I was getting out of the shower. The answering machine was just picking up as I grabbed the receiver of my new cordless phone. I walked outside my window to the rooftop of the neighboring building. This was my prized sundeck. I had recently moved from the apartment on Fifteenth Street and Eighth to a giant tenement apartment on Rivington Street with eight other people. We could just open the window and walk right out. I used the rooftop as a patio for sunbathing, vegan barbeques, and a daytime office.

A good friend and new roommate was calling. We started bantering, which led to us make fun of one of our other roommates, a mutual friend we loved. But you'd have thought he was our archenemy by the sound of our conversation. I suppose we didn't yet know how to express our true feelings.

As my friend and I joked, the answering machine recorded our conversation. We were oblivious. After about forty-five minutes of cruel comedy, we hung up and went about our days. When our other roommate got home, he checked the machine for messages and discovered our recording. He listened to it and was crushed.

When he confronted me, I tried to defend myself by saying that we'd been joking and that he joked the same way. But he was hurt to his core, and I didn't blame him. I was a fool, and our friendship was ruined. He moved out of the apartment, and I was left with self-loathing. This was a tragic lesson.

Soon after, the band went out of town for a mini tour, and I returned to reading the *Dhammapada*. I opened it to the following verses:

> Verse 231: Guard against evil deeds, control your body. Giving up evil deeds, cultivate good deeds.

> Verse 232: Guard against evil speech, control your speech. Giving up evil speech, cultivate good speech.

Verse 233: Guard against evil thoughts, control
your mind. Giving up evil thoughts, cultivate
good thoughts.

Verse 234: The wise are controlled in deed, they
are controlled in speech, they are controlled in
thought. Indeed, they are perfectly self-controlled.

I realized I had used evil speech and was reaping the rewards. Later, I opened a book of quotations that I used for songwriting inspiration to a quote from Socrates: "Strong minds discuss ideas. Average minds discuss events. Weak minds discuss people."

I was a weak mind.

My straight-edge, clean-living, clean-diet, juice-fasting lifestyle took toxins out of my body. But if my thoughts were toxic, I would be forced to speak defiled words, just like the Buddhists say. As vices or a poor diet weaken the body, there are thoughts that weaken the mind.

"Guard against defiled thoughts, control your mind," says the Buddha.

Critical speech, gossip, and jokes that magnified the faults of others were toxic mental behavior—and I was poisoning myself and spreading that poison to others. I didn't want to be that person, but I didn't know how to change my thoughts.

At the bookstore I read about Indian monks called mauna babas who make vows of silence, understanding how much damage words can cause. They don't want to create bad karma (like I did) by idle, foolish speech, gossip, and criticism, so they make vows not to speak at all. I wondered if I should be a mauna baba.

I also had a sense that specific literature was finding me at crucial times in my life. I'd jot down notes about my personal realizations so I could transform my character. If the notes were similar, I'd cluster them and then turn them into a song. Sometimes these notes would sit in notebooks for years before becoming songs. The notes I took during this period of my life became the song "In Praise of Others":

> Well, it's hard to glorify others due to my
> > intense pride
> Even amongst friends you'll find I sit and criticize
> It's what I do best, it's how I forget my actual size
> A leash that ties me to this world
>
> Yeah, a wicked mind brought me to this world,
> > Lord, please help me move forward
> I've been guilty so long, I know that I'm wrong,
> > please help me sing this song in praise of others
> In praise of others
> In praise of others
> In praise of others
>
> Can I glorify others, my sisters or my brothers,
> > or anyone else?
> Each fault that I find with you I find tenfold
> > in myself
> Envy, a disease, it's inside of me
> But I'm the loser in the end
>
> Yeah, a wicked mind brought me to this world, Lord,
> > please help me move forward
> I've been guilty so long, I know that I'm wrong,
> > please help me sing this song in praise of others
> In praise of others
> In praise of others
> In praise of others

I should have blamed myself
Instead of everyone else

But God forbid they find fault with me, we're
    instant enemies
How dare I see myself honestly as others may see?
A proud fool, I turn away, won't hear what they say,
    it might benefit me
And I remain tied in this net of pride,
    but I wanna be free

Yeah, a wicked mind brought me to this world,
    Lord, please help me move forward
I've been guilty so long, I know that I'm wrong,
    please help me sing this song in praise of others
In praise of others
In praise of others
In praise

I faced a problem with responsible speech. Words can heal, or words can hurt, and this seemed to be a stumbling block in my life. Like a rain-cloud, which at a certain point gets too heavy to hold all the water within, the themes that appeared again and again in my life would eventually pour out of me and into a song. Sometimes it would happen immediately and spontaneously. Some, like this one, took years.

*   *   *

I decided to take a course on Ayurvedic medicine with Bhagavat. The classes were crowded. He showed photos of his bodily transformation before and after adopting healthy habits. The class built on the lessons I learned from that first exam: Health was not merely about what you ate; it was also about when and what to eat according to your body's constitution. A health regimen was like a maintenance program. I learned many valuable practices, such as self-massage, or abhyanga. I started practicing abhyanga first thing in the morning using a blend of herbs and sesame or coconut oil called mahanarayana thailam. I'd start with my feet and work my way up through my ankles and legs. Then I'd do my arms and head and place drops in all the gates of the body. This energized me, increased my appetite, made my bleached hair feel less like straw, and lubricated my skin.

Bhagavat taught me to be careful about what I put on my skin. "Your skin is your mouth," he said. "You are eating whatever you put on it. Don't put things on the skin that you wouldn't put in your mouth." This advice changed my relationship with skin products.

He also taught me the benefits of cool showers in the morning, which woke up my circulation, activated my immune system, and got me out of my sleepy mind. After I ate, I lay on my left side for a few minutes to aid my digestion. He also told me to go to bed early and rise early. But while I understood the importance of this, my lifestyle didn't support it. He also advised me to stay away from negative people, a practice I'd already come to on my own.

One day, I came to Bhagavat with a health issue. I told him that my memory was weak and I was always exhausted.

He looked at me, lovingly concerned.

"That's a problem, Ray," he said. "How old are you? Nineteen? Twenty? You should be filled with energy and sharp thinking."

He pulled out a tincture of gotu kola (Indian pennywort), chyavanprash (a jam made from Indian gooseberry), and a few other herbs that I wasn't familiar with and arranged them on the counter. Then he stared me in the eye. "Can I ask you a personal question Ray?"

"Sure." I was comfortable with him.

"It's personal. Do you mind?"

"No, Bhagavat, I don't mind. Ask me anything."

"Ray, do you have a girlfriend?"

"There's a girl I'm dating," I said.

It had only been two months since I'd broken things off with Stacia and sworn off women entirely. But I'd already started seeing someone new. The pendulum of my relationship to dating swung back and forth frequently.

"Do you see this girl a lot?"

"Well, yeah. I live near her, so we hang out at each other's apartments."

"Forgive me if this is personal, Ray, but it's part of my diagnosis."

I nodded compliantly.

"Are you sexually intimate with her?"

"Sure, all the time," I said. "Whenever we get the chance."

"All the time?" he said. "Are you kidding me? All the time! Ray, you can't do that to yourself! Seriously? No wonder you're exhausted and have a bad memory!" He scooped up all the herbs I was going to buy and put them away. "These are of no use to you until you change your habits."

"Since when is sex not good for you?" I asked. "I've been told it was extremely healthy for me. I think I have a healthy sex life!"

"Not according to Ayurvedic and Chinese medicine," he said. "For the Daoists, sex was an alchemical practice of transforming the sexual essence into qi and jing. In Ayurveda, we say too much indulgence in semen loss destroys memory and vital health. Exhaustion is common. The sukra, or the semen, is considered vital. The more you waste, the more your strength and intelligence deteriorate. They say the loss of the sukra invites death, and its preservation gives life. When conserved, it is reabsorbed into the system. All the secrets of health lie in the preservation of this vital force, Ray. When men waste it, they cannot have physical, mental, moral, or spiritual development."

I had never heard that, but I remembered Stacia and how torn I had been about sex for much of my life. The prevailing thought was that sexuality should be indulged as much as possible, and sometimes I went along with that. But I also felt that sex could be addictive, degrading, and unsatisfying. It always left me a little lonely. I had heard that all animals were sad after sex. I didn't know if it was true for everyone, but it was true for me.

This was a turning point for me. Even though I felt driven to win women over, I also knew in my heart that it wouldn't give me what I needed or deeply wanted. That became my mantra when I saw a beautiful woman: *Gorgeous, yes. But not what my heart wants.*

"Thanks Bhagavat. I hear you," I said. "I never thought about it like this, but it makes sense."

Just then, I saw that he was wearing tulasi beads, which I hadn't noticed before. They were somewhat hidden by his hair.

"Are you a Krishna devotee?" I asked.

"Yes." He smiled. "Yes, I am.

"What's up with those guys?" I asked, like I'd asked Joshua. "What's up with the guru?

"If you mean A. C. Bhaktivedanta Swami," he said, "well, I traveled with him all over India. I was with him at his bedside when he passed away in the town of Vrindavan. He was translating sacred literature even as he departed from his body. A truly liberated soul."

This moved me. After that conversation I tried to practice celibacy. I wasn't great at it. And my girlfriend wasn't into it at all. Our relationship became platonic. It was awkward. I didn't know how to move forward.

*   *   *

I was feeling a little sad, a little empty, hankering internally for something. There was a God-shaped hole in my heart, and I was trying to put things in that hole that didn't fit, like popularity and validation. I *was* popular. A singer of a band and part of a community—seemingly just what an extrovert like me needed. So why was I so lonely, even in a crowd? I walked to my reading spot at Washington Square Park. I opened up the *Bhagavad Gita* to a random verse, as if I was opening a fortune cookie to see my message of the day, and this is what I read (Chapter 5, Verse 24):

> One whose happiness is within, who is active and
> rejoices within, and whose aim is inward is actually
> the perfect mystic. He is liberated in the Supreme,
> and ultimately he attains the Supreme.

It was just what I needed to hear. I felt like I needed a partner, a companion, to make me complete. A Mrs. Right to patch up a hole or a crack. But perhaps the issue was that I was turning outside to find my wholeness. This verse told me, "Stop going out. Go within."

That didn't stop my romantic illusion that some other being would make me whole. Not long after I read this verse, I saw Jennifer at the restaurant and asked her out. She blushed and said yes, and my heart felt full. But I immediately realized that this wasn't real pleasure. It was transient pleasure, which the *Gita* also spoke about. *I shouldn't be dependent on a person or thing for my own validation and wholeness*, I thought. *Those should only come from God. Humans are fallible. Humans can die.*

I thought of my father, how he went from living, smiling, and joking to comatose in a matter of moments. People leave us and break our hearts. They get sick, or they get sick of us. Why should I be happy because Jennifer wanted to go out with me when, in a matter of moments, she could be over me, leave me, or die? Why was I looking for another person to make me complete, steady, and confident? That should come from within.

I still went out with her, but in my heart I knew it wasn't her, or any person, that I was looking for. I wanted God, love, truth, and connection. This was an inside job. I felt like a zero and was trying to find another person out there to make me whole, to make me one—one with God and one with myself. But dragging another zero into my life wouldn't do it. Zero plus zero never equals one. It equals zero.

I realized that I had nothing to offer anyone until I became spiritually connected—until I knew who I was and why I was there. How dare I make a person my God or become a parasite on another lost being! It wasn't fair. Yet in the past I had fallen in love with others I thought might save me. What romantic bubbles these spiritual truths were popping! I decided that relationships were secondary. I wanted to fall in love with my higher power first.

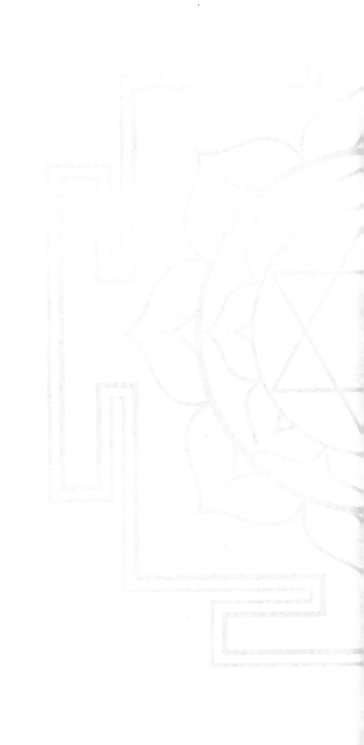

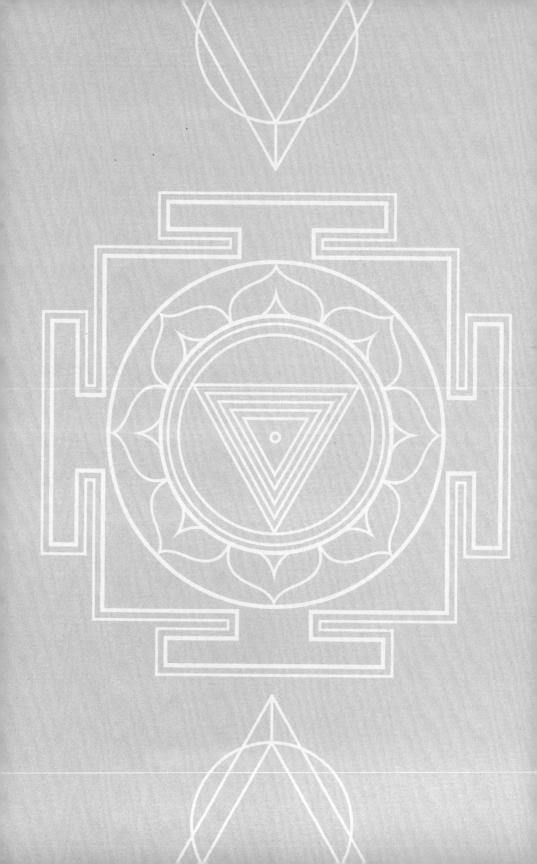

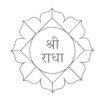

CHAPTER 5

DEEPENING SPIRITUAL CONNECTIONS

It had been a year of conscious, selective vegetarianism. Well, pesca-tarianism. I still ate fish. To curb my cravings and remind me of the cruelty of the meat industry, I trained myself to see burgers as beings, pigs as people. But I just couldn't give up eating fish. Fishing was sacred to me, a part of my childhood when life was easier, carefree, a time when I'd call my friend Tim early in the morning and say, "Let's skip school and go fishing."

Tim never needed much coaxing. Neither did I. I loved rising early before anyone was awake, slipping out of the house. Walking two and a half miles up the road seemed like walking out of civilization. I crossed over barbed-wire fences and walked through the cornfields of the Parks's farm, careful not to let neighbors or the farmer see me. There, over the first hill, hidden behind a long line of juniper and maple trees, was the sweetest pond—clean to swim and fish in and untouched by the outside world. It was my secret place. My own private world. I spent many mornings talking to that pond and the trees. I felt like I had a relationship with them all. I greeted the sun as it rose and felt it dissipate the early morning fog. The warmth of the sun affirmed my choices. A voice told me that being immersed in nature would be a better education than anything I could learn in junior high school. I started to live life based on two of my favorite books: *Huckleberry Finn* and *Walden*.

I now call it transcendental hooky. I never looked at fishing as doing something wrong or breaking rules. I ate what I caught. It was food. A fuel. A necessity. I started contemplating life and journaling on these trips. Sometimes, my more responsible mind would ask questions: *Why are you skipping school today? You could get into trouble. There's a test coming up on Tuesday! Don't be a fool!* But I ignored it.

As I lay on the tall grass with daisies around my ears, the scent of cedar, wildflowers, and dry grass was intoxicating. Every time I doubted my choices, I started my rebuttal something like this: *How many people can you name from the 1400s? A few? Twenty at most? If you're a history teacher, perhaps a hundred? But there were millions living during those times. They had real lives. They felt significant. They fell in love. They got their hearts broken. They gave birth and watched loved ones die. And then it ended, and perhaps there were three generations of family members within a hundred-year span, all thinking they were so important. But they weren't. They were tiny and insignificant, like these blades of grass. The 1400s weren't that long ago. They were nothing in the history of time. Those names and faces are erased. Who will remember or give a damn in a hundred years that I skipped school and went fishing?*

I'd lie on my back and feel secure in my insecurity, knowing that I, too, was as tiny as a blade of grass, an insignificant fraction of something much bigger than myself. I felt no guilt or shame. I felt like an honest philosopher. With the breeze in my hair and the rest of the world off in its busyness, I felt like a free man.

Those days felt wholesome, natural, and organic—a world away from New York, a world away from now. Youth of Today was touring the

United States, performing in disgusting nightclubs and bars that reeked of beer and cigarettes. That was our daily fragrance, and I was over it. I was sick of seeing bathroom stalls with graffiti drawn all over them—genitals, curses, sex, swastikas. I was sick of toilets with no seats, no doors, and urine all over the place, like we were in a human barn. I was sick of holes punched in walls. As much as I loved this music, the atmosphere was depressing. I often dreamed about Parks Pond and my days as a teenager.

One day on tour I told Mike Judge, our drummer at the time, about my childhood sacred space. I said that when this tour was over, we should go on a camping trip there. We could visit my mom in Connecticut and stay up at the pond, away from all the mess of dirty punk rock nightclubs. We could sleep under the stars and live off the land. Berries would be in season—tasty, nutritious blackcaps—and violets, dandelions, and plantain grew everywhere. Not to mention all the fish we would catch. Mike agreed. He was just as grossed out by the punk rock scene as I was. We were exhausted, and he, having grown up on a farm in rural New Jersey, appreciated my desire to reconnect with the land.

It started off beautifully. A gorgeous day. We hiked up from my childhood home carrying as little as possible. The water table was high and the spillover from the dammed falls was loud and exciting.

I want my kids to grow up like this! I thought. *This would be the best thing I could give them.* Everything was in full bloom. Nothing had changed since junior high! I inhaled the familiar perfume of meadow and forest. Nature's incense. It felt so therapeutic.

I was here again at my private Walden Pond. It meant escaping the material world. It meant diving into my inner self. It meant being connected with nature, something I had missed since moving to New York City and touring with my band. It was an anchor for sanity, calm, and connection in my life. If giving up fishing and consuming fish would mean giving up that state of being, I couldn't do that yet.

But something had shifted in me over the past year. I hadn't given up meat for health reasons, like many others. My choice came from not wanting to cause unnecessary pain. I kept that message as a personal mantra. *Minimize pain to others.* This, I felt, was an ethical choice. I'd been challenged again and again, but now I'd made it a year without meat.

This opening of my heart was about to ruin my fishing trip.

I struggled with the basics. The *real* basics. I didn't want to put a worm on the hook! It was torturous. When I was a kid, fishing with Tim, I got a thrill out of shaking my Hula Popper across the still water with a delicate snap of my wrist so my lure would resemble a helpless frog or bug. There was another thrill as the bass ran with my bait. There was the excitement of the fight. There was the silly feeling of strength as I set the hook, let the drag out, and reeled it in. I say *silly* because it's not like I was fishing for an orca. It was a fish the size of my hand, or forearm at best. Big deal, I fooled a little fish. But there *was* and *is* a power in controlling and capturing, an instinctual feeling of being a conqueror. It used to fuel my ego, creating a peculiar if not primal feeling of dominance.

Now, when I poked the worm with the sharpened hook and saw it struggle for its life, I thought, *What the hell am I doing creating so much pain for this guy? How can I be oblivious of this being's struggle?* I stared at my palm, holding the worms . . . and I turned a part of my heart off. I continued the task at hand, berating myself. *This is fishing! This is a good thing! This is normal. You are* not *in a dirty punk rock bathroom. It's a Norman Rockwell painting. Native Americans did it. Sailors did it. Kids and their dads do it. Everybody does it. It's healthy. It makes* me *healthy. This is a good thing!*

I cast my bait out into the pond using worms on a treble hook with a floating bobber. It didn't take long before that bobber was hit and descended underwater. The adrenaline flew through my veins, and the sound of the drag of my line, on my ultralight spinning tackle, excited my senses. This happened four times within an hour. I held and examined each fish and looked at them. There was an artistic beauty in those largemouth bass and bluegills. An intelligence. These were beings that I had just snatched from their homes. I put them on a stringer—a twinelike piece of nylon going through the gills and out of their mouths. Then I secured them to an underwater branch and put them back in the water so they would stay fresh.

I caught another largemouth bass. The fight was strong for my rod and reel, and he broke water in the most beautiful way. The thrill of domination came over me, as if I was harpooning Moby Dick. I reeled him in, the biggest fight yet. When it was over, I picked him up only to realize he had all three prongs of the treble hook caught in his mouth, one of them going through the top of his palate, then puncturing and coming out of his eye socket.

There was no easy way to remove the hook from this fish without killing or severely maiming it. And that's exactly what happened. I stood there holding this mangled fish, still alive. I stared at it as it flapped about desperately, most likely filled with utter dread and anxiety. I took a deep breath. This had never happened to me when I was a teenager. I didn't think twice about ripping a hook out of a fish's mouth. Now I stood looking at this guy, as devastated as if I had lost a family member.

I looked over at Mike and said, "I can't do this anymore. I don't have to do this to enjoy the pond, the sky, and the trees. I don't have to pluck every flower or cage every leopard to appreciate their beauty. Beauty can exist without me having to control it, dominate it, and possess it. This part of my life is over—but I'm going to keep the forest, sky, and pond. There's plenty of food out here to eat."

We made some porridge we'd brought, stir-fried some wild greens, and ate a few handfuls of berries. Then we rested under the stars.

*　　*　　*

Exactly nine blocks up from my apartment on Fifteenth Street was the Sivananda Ashram, a center for Vedic spiritual growth that was founded by the late Swami Sivananda. I went there frequently to practice yoga and pranayama and immerse myself in the wall of books he'd written. Swami Sivananda was a strict follower of the Vedic path, giving up his life as a physician to be a parivrajakacharya sannyasi, or traveling mendicant, before finally settling down on the bank of the river Ganges in Rishikesh, India, in 1936. This is where he started the Divine Life Society, a Hindu spiritual organization that now has branches all over the world.

He was a prolific writer on topics such as Vedanta, bhakti, karma yoga, and jnana yoga, among so many others. He wrote two hundred books in all. All of them said "free to replicate as one likes" on the inside jacket. I would make myself comfortable on the floor and pick through these books like I was spending a day in the library. The people working there didn't care. They probably thought I'd join their organization, so they were encouraging. I thought these wisdom teachings would be a valuable source for writing lyrics, like the *Bhagavata Gita* was, since wisdom lasts forever. I was always looking for ideas for songs.

I picked up a book called *Japa Yoga* by Swami Sivananda. *Japa* is the recitation of mantras on beads, and I was curious about its efficacy. I read the following:

> There is a Shakti or power in every word. If you utter
> the word "excreta" or "urine" when your friend is
> taking his meals, he may at once vomit his food.

> If you think of "Garam Pakoda," "hot Pakoda" (fried
> delicacies), your tongue will get salivation. When
> anyone suddenly shouts "Scorpion! Scorpion!",
> "Snake! Snake!", you at once apprehend the scorpion
> or the snake and jump in fright. When anyone calls
> you a "donkey" or an "ass," you are annoyed and you
> show anger. If anyone says, "You are a nice person,"

you smile. When such is the power of the names
of the ordinary things of this world, what tremendous power should there be in the Name of God!
God is the completion or the fullness of existence.
Hence, the Name which denotes Him, too, is full
and perfect. Therefore, the power of the Name of
God is incalculable, for it is the height or the zenith
of power. The Name of God can achieve anything.
There is nothing impossible for it. It is the means
to the realization of God Himself.

I thought, *I need some japa in my life!* This planted the seed of interest
in mantras and sounds to transform consciousness.

* * *

I'd go back and forth between the Sivananda Ashram and the Integral Yoga
Institute, which was also near my apartment. During this time, I finally
figured out how to do a headstand and stay in that position peacefully for
twenty breaths. The practice of movement and conscious breathing had a
radical effect on me, and I witnessed my body and consciousness change.
I always left yoga feeling a little more relaxed, unlike a workout at the gym,
where I'd be exhausted and wired. Like the Sivananda Ashram, Integral
Yoga had a large bookstore inside it, which I also loitered in.

One day, I was reading a book by Swami Sivananda, and I found a verse
that asked where we get our pleasure from. Was it tangible pleasure or was
it the pleasure of the ego? It said that our dharma should give us worth,
not the things of this world. This stuck with me because I had already been
thinking about love and lust and how physical beauty, sexual pleasure, and
romantic relationships played into that, and this seemed similar.

I started to think about something I got a lot of pleasure from: my collection of rare punk singles and LPs. Because punk bands broke up often and didn't press that many units, the records quickly became collector items. We lived in a major city, so Porcell and I would scour the stores to find rare treasures to add to our collections. After I started Revelation Records with Jordan, we'd press limited-run records merely so I could trade with record stores to increase my collection. Records are delicate and can scratch and warp easily, so I treated them with great care, keeping them sealed in plastic and only playing the actual albums on cassette. I loved all of these bands, but this was sonic materialism.

Where do I get my pleasure from if I'm not playing *the records?* I thought, staring into space at the bookstore. The heady, masculine scent of agarwood incense unfurled beneath a cartoonlike poster of Lord Shiva. *I guess there's pleasure in the search, almost like a treasure hunt to find the rare records. But it's not a tangible pleasure. It's in my mind. The pleasure comes when I show them to someone else who collects them.* The last time I did this, I marched home to my apartment with ten Bad Brains singles—incredibly rare. An almost impossible find. And I'd found ten! I discovered them at a little-known record store that I frequented, hidden on a shelf behind the counter. I felt like a California miner discovering gold nuggets. I walked in the door and blew Porcell's mind.

In that moment, I clenched my jaw as I came to terms with a serious realization: This wasn't tangible pleasure at all. *These records are merely ornaments for my ego.* In the same way that someone might show off a sports car or a Rolex, I showed off my records. This made me feel cooler—better—than other people. But it was just stuff. Stuff couldn't give me joy, but living in Buddha consciousness or Christ consciousness could.

Over the next year, I started throwing these records out into the crowd at our performances. Some people thought I was foolish, but it was one of the most liberating things I had ever done. I was throwing away an illusion, things that would ultimately get stored in a closet until another collector came over. I didn't regret it. I threw away part of an old identity, a skin that needed to be shed.

*   *   *

Although I was working at the restaurant, I needed more money and found a club downtown that was different from the Tunnel. Instead of being a raging disco, it hosted world music, and it sold not only alcohol but also carrot juice and other nonalcoholic beverages. Pretty progressive! It was a place to go out and enjoy the world, but it wasn't solely based on intoxication. I felt like the universe had brought me here to let go of the degrading club life and give me a higher alternative. After I was hired, that place became my new oasis.

This time, I didn't want to be on the floor. I worked behind the scenes in the offices during the evening, doing odd jobs and assisting a coworker named Maryanne. I sat next to her. She was about thirty-five and attractive, and a spiritual seeker like me—pretty much everyone there was.

One day we started talking about vegetarianism. I broke into my usual rant that animals are spiritual beings and should be respected as such. "We shouldn't take their lives to satisfy the whim of our palates," I said. "We should treat them with dignity and care."

She countered my argument, saying some spiritual books, like the Bible, say that humans have dominion over animals. I argued that parents had dominion over their children, but that didn't mean they should beat or abuse them. *Dominion,* I argued, meant to steward, care for, and love. She agreed. I think I converted her to vegetarianism that evening. I was on a mission. I felt like every person claiming they were spiritual needed to complete that logic by adopting a cruelty-free diet.

"Well, it's no wonder James hired you," she said. "I think you two must be very close."

"Who's James?"

"Wait, you don't know James?" she asked. "How did you get this job? I thought you must be one of his students or protégés."

"No," I said. "I got the job through an ad in the *Village Voice*."

"He's the owner here, and a powerful spiritual being," she said. "He teaches us how to meditate. We go to his house for sacred prayers and rituals. He has the ability to manifest whatever he wants. He's fabulously rich! But he's also difficult to figure out. If he desires something, he gets it. But he never takes credit. He said it's the divine spirit working through him. I can't believe you got a job here *randomly!*" Her face was full of excitement. "James must have willed you to be here!"

I was intrigued. Who was this guy? *Had* I been willed here? I knew my life was turning more toward the spirit. I went home that night excited. I prayed. *The spirit is calling me*, I thought. *Because I'm desiring it, spirit is pulling me forward.*

No one in my band related to this. They didn't want to hear that the spirit was calling me. They felt that I was slipping. That maybe I was losing my mind. Or, at the very least, that I was veering off-brand. After all, Porcell and I had helped create the image and philosophy of straight edge. We kept it simple: We were clean-cut; we weren't into drugs or other intoxication; we were strict vegetarians. It was a different brand—though no less alternative in those days—than punk rock and hardcore. It was a huge pill to swallow for teenagers who were accustomed to sex, drugs, and buzz-saw guitars, yet they were swallowing it. By this point, tens of thousands of teens around the world were opting in to this lifestyle. We had started receiving international fan mail. We'd never planned for it to be a movement. It used to be *our* thing, but now it a was thing in and of itself.

And so my bandmates probably felt some responsibility to the scene. They felt that our brand was simple, and the spiritual stuff didn't really fit into that. Christ consciousness. Oneness. The Buddha-nature. The

Bhagavad Gita. Sadhus. Swamis. Lamas. Our fans didn't relate to it. When my banter started leaning toward the spiritual in interviews or onstage, my bandmates were quick to drag the conversation back to the band's basic tenets. Sometimes they'd say, "Well, that's Ray's thing." But the spiritual pull was a genuine current in my life, and my philosophy didn't start and stop with abstaining from drugs. The straight-edge principles of self-control were incredibly important, but they were the threshold to something more esoteric and metaphysical.

When I came into work the next day, the club was blaring beautiful African dance music, and I squirmed my way through the crowd of rhythmically moving bodies to the back office. I sat down next to Maryanne. She told me that she kept thinking about something I'd said the night before, that *dominion* means to care for, not to exploit. We started talking about what it meant to be spiritual, how even *acting* spiritual can be a manifestation of ego. We shared the books we were reading, like *Autobiography of a Yogi, Jonathan Livingston Seagull,* and *Siddhartha.* She was a kindred spirit.

Throughout the conversation, she mentioned James—"James *always* says that!" and "James recommended I do that" and "James is *really* into that." I just nodded.

A woman burst into the room, almost spilling her carrot juice. "Where's James? Is he here?" she asked in a Long Island accent. "Last night I saw an angel! I kid you not! I need to know what that means. I need to know if it's a dream or if it was real. I *need* to talk to James!"

Maryanne introduced me to Monica, who also worked in the club. She told Monica about our conversation and my quest to practice nonviolence through a nonviolent diet.

"That's so profound!" said Monica. "I'm macrobiotic. James must *love* you! Where did he find you?" She turned to Maryanne "Where the hell did James find this kid?"

As I'd told Maryanne the night before, I said that I didn't know him. And like Maryanne, Monica was shocked and said that James must have manifested me. Now I was even more intrigued. This guy was a guru, a person you could ask about angels, someone who taught meditation, *and* attracted wealth to him by will?

The next night, I was in the office late with Maryanne when a tall, Jesus-looking man entered, probably in his late forties. He had shoulder-length, sandy-blond hair, a beard, and a mustache. He wore a white suit and tan cowboy boots.

"Hello. I'm James," he said, eyes twinkling. He placed his hands in namaste, and I returned the gesture.

"James," Maryanne said, "this is my new assistant, Ray. He's a singer in a band that's against drugs and alcohol. He has deep spiritual insight into animals."

James approached me slowly and dramatically. He sat down, getting awkwardly close to me, never breaking his gaze. "Explain your insight into animals. I'd love to hear." He gave me his full attention, his face that of a humble student.

So, I started preaching to him like I preached to everyone else, speaking quietly but firmly. James listened intently, and I felt a calming quiet spread over the room.

"Mahatma Gandhi said a culture can be judged by how it treats its animals," I said, "I want to create a new culture of spiritual compassion—"

"*Freeze!*" James suddenly screamed, cutting me off. I froze. Then he paused and was quiet. I was scared. "Look at your hand, Ray," he said, "Look. At. Your. Hand!"

I looked at my frozen outstretched hand. "What?"

He grabbed my hand. "Don't move your hand, Ray!" he screamed. Then he whispered again. "Jnana mudra. Your thumb is touching your pointer finger. Your hand was in jnana mudra when you were speaking to me.

Jnana means knowledge. Knowledge is possessing your body. When you speak, it's as if spirit is speaking. Just look at your hand."

It *was* in jnana mudra. Maybe I was a mystic and I didn't even realize it!

"Yes, you were sent here." James got up, shook off his intensity, paced for a moment and moved his head back and forth. "We have great work to do, Ray." Then he walked out of the room. Monica and Maryanne looked at me as if I was the Chosen One, but they said nothing.

On my walk home, I started thinking about how God sent people to educate you when you were ready. I was so ready. The material world was becoming painful. My father was still in a coma—something I still could barely even speak about. My band was getting bigger, and because of it, life was growing more complex.

I needed a teacher.

*   *   *

I felt fortunate. I was able to make my own music. I had been invited to play all over the United States. There was an audience who were into us and our message. There were dedicated fans that knew our lyrics. I was paid to play, something most musicians could never say. People appreciated our records, followed our philosophy of clean living, and adopted the principles we espoused. We had support around the world.

In one sense, for a young person making music it was a dream come true. But with magnified pleasure comes magnified pain. I didn't think I was alone in feeling the pain of success. People in many careers felt such things. First, there was the pain of fear—fear of losing our success. Then there was the pain of the ego that came with success. Finally, the sad nature of human envy and competition that plagues all of us.

The Buddha said, "Do not overrate what you have received, nor envy others. He who envies others does not obtain peace of mind." I could feel that I was losing peace of mind as our material success grew. I was operating out of fear, overly concerned about what fans thought of us, what our reviews were like, and whether people liked our records.

I wanted our fame to grow. At the same time, there were bands that we'd supported who weren't as big as us but who were now publicly speaking ill of us. I became envious of other bands, and I could feel the envy of others. Envy truly is the art of counting another's blessings and forgetting one's own. It's insatiable. Exhausting. All my spiritual readings and lifestyle choices had created a new metric for happiness, which shined a light on the futility of material success. The great masters spoke of happiness separate from ego, envy, competition, and pride. Would I ever be able to achieve that?

One day I was in the office alone when James walked in and sat down. He looked at me as if he was reading my mind. It was a little weird, but also cool and mystical.

"I've got something for you," he said. He pulled out a piece of paper and wrote down the letters M-A-L-A. "This is a mala," he said. "They are for recitation of sacred sounds called mantras. I'm going to give you a mantra today, and it will help you understand that you are divine and you are God."

He reached into his shoulder bag and pulled out a beautiful set of carved brown beads.

"This is your mala. Repeat after me," he said slowly, as if I were a child. "Om mani."

"Om mani," I said.

"Padme hum."

"Padme hum," I repeated.

"Om mani padme hum."

"Om mani padme hum," I repeated again.

"Om mani padme hum, om mani padme hum," he said.

"Om mani padme hum, om mani padme hum," I said.

Then he started repeating the mantra really fast, like an LP playing at 78 rpm. It sounded like gibberish. I was sort of stunned, but I tried to imitate him in that same fast, high-pitched voice. If anybody else had been around I would have felt foolish. But in that room with James, I was all in. I'd do anything to have peace of mind, and I knew that mantras were powerful and transformational.

When we stopped, I asked him what the mantra meant.

"It means, Ray, that *you* are the jewel in the lotus," he said cryptically.

"Uh, well what does *that* mean?" I asked.

"*You* are the God you are looking for. You are that Divinity. You are that Almighty. You are that Mystic. It isn't out there. It's inside."

"If I'm God, then why do I make foolish choices again and again?" I asked. "What kind of God acts like that?"

"There is a path to get out of that cycle," James said. "Chant these mantras and awaken your Buddha-nature. It's already in you, but you've forgotten. I've been sent, Ray, to wake you up!"

*   *   *

Alone in my room, I practiced the mantra James—whom I dubbed Guru James in my mind—had given me. I'd just moved to a new apartment in Williamsburg, Brooklyn, with Porcell and Alex. I closed the door to my room and chanted. My roommates heard me and thought I'd lost my mind. All they heard was high-pitched chirping through my closed door. I was their friend, but now I was howling mantras in the other room.

I didn't think I was going too far, though. James hadn't made this up. Mantras were as old as time. I'd read books on chanting mantras for wealth, health, progeny, longevity, even love. I knew the sounds that came out of our mouths were powerful and transformational. I knew yogis used mantras, or codified sounds, to create inner change. I knew from being a musician that sound could cause people to love or hate. I also knew that there were sounds that lingered in the mind in the form of thoughts or self-talk. Sometimes those sounds served us, and sometimes they brought us down. So I knew that mantras must do *something*. I just wasn't sure what.

*   *   *

There was a small minority of full-blown Nazis in the music scene. They didn't always show up to shows—and they were never welcome—but when they did, they always brought chaos. Nazis were violent and provocative. Why did they come to shows? Because whether you were a Nazi, an extreme-left anarcho-communist, a punk with a spiked mohawk, or a straight-edge skater, you were a freak. And in the 1980s, freaks found other freaks.

In my songs and onstage I was always outspoken against racism. I borrowed my philosophy from wisdom literature. We are all spiritual beings, and the body is our shell, merely a vehicle for spirit. Why hate? We are basically all the same underneath the costume. I had to be careful to hate the racism and not the racist. As the Bible said, hate the sin not the sinner. Once you hate the sinner, you've become hateful. And that meant you lost the game, becoming the thing you hated. After all, anyone can change at any moment. If we are beings of love, then compassion and forgiveness are key ingredients—and can transform the world.

One day on tour, my outspokenness got me in trouble. I was watching an opening band, and a skinhead came up to me and elbowed me in the face. Of course, this led to an all-out war with my band, who started to collect pool sticks and bar stools. I didn't realize the guy was part of a gang, not just one random kid with an attitude. Thankfully, the bouncers broke things up before it got too crazy.

We took the stage, but there was still a lot of anger and hate in the room. I read from my lyrics and spoke about unity. I spoke about hate breeding more hate. About how nobody ends up winning. Sometimes, my speaking up like this brought about understanding, but other times there was just too much fury in the air.

I wrote a song called "Prejudice" about racism and other forms of shallow thinking. The song spoke to so many people. I received thousands of letters about it. Kids shared how this song in particular had saved them during critical times of their lives and helped them deal with proselytizing racists. Unfortunately, the song also provoked racists to call me out, climb on stage, assault me, or organize an attack on the band, which is what happened with the skinhead who elbowed me.

The message held, though. Hate does not win. Hate causes hate. Love is louder. Love is the winner.

*   *   *

Youth of Today got offered a gig in Washington, D.C.. The band never got hotels. Ever. We just slept wherever we could. In the van. Random fans' houses. Promoters' houses. Lawns. Squats. Porcell and I still strongly believed that the universe would provide for us, and we continued to accept whatever we got, which kept us tolerant, humble, and flexible for whatever we received. It was great sadhu training and later made monk life a natural transition for me.

In Washington, D.C., we stayed at the house of a friend in the punk scene who lived with a bunch of eclectic, ultraliberal, free-thinking people. We didn't know them. It was always awkward walking into a house full of people we didn't really know and trying to make ourselves at home. The two-story house was run-down, but that was expected of a rental shared by twelve teenagers and twentysomethings. Punk posters and flyers decorated the walls. Thrashy music played loudly at 10 a.m. (not my cup of tea). A few random cats prowled the kitchen countertops, licking the margarine.

We walked into the crowded kitchen, and after some brief introductions, I asked if I could use the bathroom. They directed me upstairs, and I quickly shot up the steps, opened one of the doors, and saw something that made me stop in my tracks. It wasn't the fact that it was a room with nothing in it—not a single piece of furniture, not a curtain on the window, not a picture on the wall. It was the fact that, sitting in the middle of the floor, was a naked man about twenty-seven years old with a Ulysses S. Grant beard. He was building a small wooden box. He had a screwdriver. Measuring tape. A hand saw. And there he sat, nude. Creating.

"Oh, I'm sorry. I'm looking for a bathroom," I said, feeling like I'd barged in on something intimate.

He looked up nonchalantly. "Bathroom's over there." He pointed to one of the doors.

I said nothing as I headed for the bathroom. I didn't want to seem unenlightened, close-minded, or judgmental of the fact that there was a big naked man in the center of an empty room. I sat on the toilet with my grandest, most broad-minded thoughts. *Big deal. A guy is sitting there naked, building a box. What's wrong with that? Why can't people do things naked? Why am I so judgmental?* Traveling around the world and meeting a wide variety of people is always a good way to step out of one's comfort zone. Here was another opportunity.

When I came out of the bathroom, he was struggling with a Phillips-head screwdriver.

"Hey man, what are you doing?" I asked.

"Putting this damn box together," he said. He looked frustrated.

"Just curious," I said, "why you are building that box . . . nude?"

He stopped, apparently disturbed. He put down the screwdriver. "What do you expect me to wear?" he asked.

Good question. It caught me off guard.

"Uh . . . I don't know," I said, stumbling, "pants?"

"Why?" he said sharply. "Because somebody told us to wear pants? Why not a robe like a Roman or a Greek? Why not a skirt like a Scottish man?

Don't you understand, man? All your concepts of clothing have been programmed into you by the media. You are just a helpless puppet in the hands of Madison Avenue selling you shit." He was clearly vexed. "It's not just media—it's culture. One time in history, men wore white wigs. Women wore massive dresses. Men wore buckled shoes, knee socks. Why don't *you* wear any of those? I'll tell you why . . . because you're a *puppet boy.* But not me. I'll wear whatever I *want* to wear. Or I'll wear nothing at all!" He went back to building.

I felt awkward. I was in this guy's house and now he was angry with me. I hadn't meant to pick a fight with him, and the last thing I wanted to do was get in a physical or verbal altercation with a naked man holding tools. He'd made a good point. Why *did* we dress the way we did? Were we just products of conditioning and programming? Why did culture change fashions every decade? What was our authentic choice? Who were we before we were programmed? What would we be like unprogrammed? I had a lot to think about.

I went back down into the kitchen to join my bandmates, and we sat around having lemonade and coffee. The man came downstairs holding his box. He wasn't nude anymore, but my bandmates were still stunned. He was wearing a ragged secondhand dress and tennis shoes. The rest of the band sort of froze as he made casual conversation with us. But at that point, I just rolled with it.

*   *   *

When I got back from Washington, I went to the club to work, hoping, of course, to see Guru James. I went to the bar and got my carrot juice mixed with apple. The live band was playing a type of music that combined African drums and keyboards. I went into the office and sat at my desk. Then Guru James walked in. He had on his white suit and cowboy boots, but today he seemed sullen.

"Ray, we have great work to do," he said firmly.

His tone took me aback. I wanted to trust him because he seemed like a spiritual authority. I definitely wasn't a spiritual authority, and I'd heard that when you're searching, the universe will send you a teacher. Was Guru James my teacher? A teacher who saw some great potential in me? Could I trust him?

He gave me a silver and turquoise case. It was the size of my hand and ornately decorated. I felt like he was handing me a magical key.

"I want you to have these and use them with your mantra meditation."

I opened the treasure chest, and my heart dropped. Inside were dried mushrooms, and I immediately understood that they were hallucinogenic. I had never done hallucinogens. I had never been interested in any recreational drugs. I had helped create an entire movement around *not* doing such things, and now this person whom I (along with the rest of the nightclub) considered a spiritual authority was handing me a box of them.

"I don't do any recreational drugs, James," I said. "I'm into the idea that the yoga system speaks about. I believe in controlling your mind and senses to find inner peace."

"Yes, I understand," he said after a beat. "But these *aren't* recreational. They're spiritual. They give you access to higher realms and dimensions that you cannot perceive on this plane. They've been used by aboriginal people for generations, and they are a shortcut to your spiritual awakening."

"Why would God make us take something external to find our internal self?" I politely inquired.

"God gives us tools to use, medicines to heal our troubled minds."

I *had* read of traditions that used psychedelics for metaphysical purposes. I had read works by Carlos Castaneda, Dr. Richard Alpert (Ram Dass), and Timothy Leary, and they often gave some credibility to psychedelics as a gateway to spirituality. But I was never exposed to them in that regard. Anyone I knew who had done LSD or mushrooms used them recreationally. A good friend of mine in high school jumped in front of a moving train on LSD. I had written songs about how experimenting with my mind was not for me. I wanted *clarity* of mind.

But I challenged myself. *What do I know of sacred traditions?* I thought. *What do I know of mantras? Herbal medicines? Metaphysical realities?* I was an infant in spiritual circles, and James seemed to be doing something right with his life. He was respected and materially successful. He had insight into things I had never heard of. The only hiccup was that it went against the values that I sang about onstage.

"Ray, the desire to eliminate intoxicants from your life is a noble cause," he said. "I understand your conundrum. But you have much to learn about the ways of mystical masters."

I couldn't argue with that. I *did* have much to learn.

*　*　*

Porcell is going to kill me, I thought. *But he doesn't understand where I'm at. Nobody understands where I'm at right now.* I, of course, struggled with the decision to take mushrooms as a leader of the straight-edge community, but I felt my spiritual calling was more important and that I'd been led to James. I was not going to do this for recreational purposes, and that seemed different to me.

I locked myself in my room and started my meditation, first silently breathing, as I had learned in my yoga classes with Dharma, to clear my head of noise, fear, and resentment. Then I made an herbal tea out of the mushrooms, as if I had done it in a previous life. Next, I started chanting the mantra *om mani padme hum* on the mala James had given me. At first slow, and then high-pitched.

I was riddled with guilt. My words and lyrics spoke of sense control, and I was a leader of thousands who followed those values. I continued breathing to clear my head of those thoughts. On the other hand, I didn't give a rat's ass about what people thought about me at this point in my life. I wanted God, and if this was a way to a metaphysical realm, as James had said, then I was open to it as my highest choice.

I drank the tea.

Almost immediately, I lost control of my sensual awareness, and my consciousness started expanding and contracting. I entered another realm. Still, I maintained my chanting as I was instructed. My room, which I valued as my domain, my artistic space, my corner of the universe, started looking different. I realized that every poster on my wall, every piece of retro furniture I'd collected, all the art I had hanging, and all the details I used to decorate my space to make it mine were manifestations of my ego. My ego was desperately trying to find validation in a universe that couldn't care less. It was all I could see.

I also realized that this room was hundreds of years old. Many other families had lived here before me. People living, dying, giving birth. It was like I was watching a black-and-white movie. I started seeing the apartment building itself as temporary, a manifestation of wood and metal, plaster and paint, soon to be crumbled back into the earth. I had been thinking about painting my room, but now that seemed futile.

I felt that I had spent my life creating meaning where there was no meaning. Meaning over fashion. Over music. Over my so-called artistic insight. Over my likes and dislikes. Ray Cappo's life—with all its excitement, fear, happiness, joy, death—was a blink of an eye in the eternality of the soul.

I started seeing myself as an aging man, just another name who had lived and died in this apartment, absorbed in my own self-importance and ultimately forgotten just like everyone else.

We are all so damn self-important, I thought, shaking my head. *We're all just buying time before we die.*

Louder and louder, I heard the voices of the *Bhagavad Gita* lectures. They spoke to me thunderously: "This is all an illusion. This is all temporary.

You've been overly concerned about this dream. There's a reality waiting for you."

At that moment I lay back on the floor, stared at the ceiling, and spoke out loud to myself. "Everything those Krishna guys have told me is correct," I said. "Everything they told me is true. This material world is all temporary. How can I go on with my life now that I understand this?"

*   *   *

Not long after my mushroom trip, Youth of Today performed in Southern California. I was staying with Zack de la Rocha (who would later help form Rage Against the Machine but wasn't yet famous) at his parents' house in Irvine. Zack was a fan of Youth of Today and at one point said we'd inspired him to go vegetarian. He was seventeen, and I was twenty. He was incredibly talented, fun, and thoughtful, and we shared a liking for fast hardcore music, stage diving, and losing ourselves in the moment.

I was always looking for new vegetarian restaurants, and I knew there was a Krishna temple in Laguna Beach, about thirty-five minutes away, that had a small vegetarian café inside. So we headed there one day.

We walked into the café and peered into the mysterious temple, which was small but charming, situated a block from the Pacific Ocean. We decided to go in before we ate. We kicked off our shoes to have a glimpse of the altar and paintings. It was an old church painted brightly and tastefully, yet it didn't have the gravity and gloominess of some of the churches I had grown up in. There were no pews; it was an open checkered floor like a chessboard. There were massive paintings on the walls depicting the life of Chaitanya, the Kirtan Avatar, though I didn't know who he was at the time. The paintings were mesmerizing. We both stood and gazed at them, trying to figure out what was going on. The deities on the altar appeared foreign to me. There were five beautifully carved statues of men. Some had their hands in namaste, while others had their hands in the air.

I didn't really understand Hindu deities, but their presence was bold and beautiful. It felt holy. The temple was pretty much empty, with a library of sacred books on the shelf and a vyasasana, or seat for the speaker, with some cushions stacked up against the wall. I could smell the incense that had burned there perhaps a few hours ago. It was a sensational experience in every sense of the world. My senses were experiencing something other-worldly with the artwork, the altar, the smells, and the sounds of music and mantras playing softly in the background.

Although I was touring, writing, and recording records, my life's direction seemed confused. I was being creative, prolific, and spreading a good message, but I wanted to have depth, wisdom, and purpose. I was over being a frivolous child.

We put our shoes on and went back into the café, where we grabbed a tray and headed through the buffet, picking out salad, curried vegetables, basmati rice, some moong dal, and a small dessert.

I wondered if they would let me experience a night in the temple. A young monk walked out, and I asked him who ran the place. He pointed to an older man with light-brown hair in a tuft of a ponytail on the back of the head. The older Krishna devotee had a grave, sweet face and was wearing a hooded sweatshirt with an Indian robe. A nice combination of East meets West.

"Excuse me, are you in charge here?" I asked.

"Yes," he said, and gave me a sweet smile.

"Could I stay here overnight sometime to see what it's like? I'm visiting from New York for a while, and I'm interested in Eastern thought and spirituality."

He looked me up and down and nodded. "Yeah, sure. My name is Bada Hari. Do you want to come back tomorrow and stay overnight?"

"Sure," I said, surprised at how easy that was.

Zack and I went back to his parents' house.

"Are you sure you want to do this?" he asked.

"Yes," I said. "What's the worst that could happen?"

"Cult indoctrination maybe?" he joked.

"Kidnapping. Castration perhaps?" I added.

We laughed, and the next day he dropped me off with my small backpack at the temple door on Legion Street in Laguna Beach.

*　*　*

I met the temple elder Bada Hari, and he invited me in to help him do some work in the kitchen washing pots. I was up for anything and started washing them with vigor.

"Can I ask you a question?" I asked while he was cutting vegetables.

"Sure, Ray."

"How do you believe all this stuff? It's a big pill to swallow. God is a blue cowherd boy. There's life on other planets. There's a sun god, a moon god, a wind god . . . how are we supposed to turn off our rational minds and just accept all these fantastic stories? I mean, we're adults . . ." I trailed off, thinking I was being profound.

"What do we know, Ray?" he asked. "Seriously." He stopped cutting. "What do we actually know?" A small ant was crawling along the counter, near where he was cutting. "Do you see that ant?"

I nodded.

"Do you think that ant knows we're in a temple? Does the ant know you have blue jeans on? Or that we're a block away from the ocean? Do you think the ant knows that?"

I shook my head.

"No," he said. "It's all real though. You *are* wearing blue jeans, and we *are* in a temple, and we *are* near the ocean. But it's beyond the ant's perception to understand it, even though he's right next to us. He's right here, and he's clueless. He doesn't have the capacity to understand, even though we are right in front of him."

133

I knew where he was going with this analogy.

"We are those ants, Ray," he said. "Arrogant. We think we know everything, but we're clueless. We guess. Speculate. Come up with theories—but we're like ants. Ants with theories, trying to figure out what is beyond our sense perception. We're trying desperately to get perfect knowledge with our imperfect antlike senses. The Vedic teachings give us a clue into reality. And reality is fantastic. It's not ordinary." He paused while I digested what he said. "No one is asking you to accept those fantastic things. In Vedic teachings we are not looking for blind followers. This isn't faith-based—it's experienced-based teaching. We ask you to bring your discernment, your intelligence, your doubts . . . and then enter the experiment. So to say 'Yes, Ganesh is definitely an elephant-headed being who scribed the Vedas' might sound like blind faith. But to say he *doesn't* exist—and you *know* that for sure—that's blind doubt. How do we know? We are like ants. We do not know if Ganesh exists, and we do not know if he doesn't exist. The safest thing to say is 'He could. He *could* exist. I don't know. But he could. Because I know very little.' So I tend to focus on the things I do know."

"Like what?" I asked. "What do you actually know about this philosophy that you can say you know for sure?"

"I know it's good to control my senses instead of indulging them."

I nodded.

"I know that rising early and taking cold showers is good for my health and that meditation is good early in the morning," he said. "I know that I don't want to kill animals for food, because they suffer tremendously."

I kept nodding.

"I know that I'm not in control of my life. I have some control, but I don't have complete control. I know there's a limit to my sensory perception."

"What do you mean?"

"For example, my ears cannot hear what a dog can hear. There are colors I cannot see. My senses are limited and subjective—like the ant's. I also know that chanting has an effect on my consciousness. It affects me profoundly. This I know from experimenting with it. I know that the sounds that come out of my mouth, both negative and positive, affect me and my environment. If I gossip, it affects me. If I speak kindly, it affects me. I know that the *Gita* is a book of wisdom. I can understand that I am a spirit who has a body. I can witness my body change and see its transformations."

I started to see his point.

"So, yes. In small increments we move forward with faith, constantly questioning."

"I get it," I said, "but it's hard. I'm just filled with so much skepticism and doubt."

"Oh, you're a doubter? Discernment is good, but be careful. Doubters stay paralyzed, in business, relationships, and even their spiritual life. Use discernment. Ask questions. But be careful with too much doubting. Or if you're going to doubt"—he paused—"why not just doubt your doubts?"

I smiled. *Yes*, I thought. *Doubt my doubts.*

* * *

I was excited and nervous to stay overnight. I packed my sleeping bag, a small towel, a toothbrush, and some coconut oil and walked over to the men's ashram, which was an apartment down the street. It was stark and underwhelming, with a few bunk beds, a painting of some male and female gods—I wasn't sure who—and some sacred books on a shelf. It was dark when I got there, and a few monks were already asleep. I was quietly shown to my bed. I crept inside, unrolled my sleeping bag, and fell fast asleep.

I was awakened at 4 a.m. when people started hurrying about to get dressed—morning services started at 4:30. I planned to go, but I figured I had half an hour to kill. I sat up in my bunk and grabbed the *Bhagavad Gita* from a shelf. Meanwhile, a few monks hustled in and out of the bathroom, draping themselves in their robes and applying sacred clay to their forehead. The clay was in a bar the size of a Milky Way, but it was tan and hard, like stone. They'd pour a few drops of water in their palm and mix the clay bar into the water, making a soft, creamy paste. With delicate accuracy, they'd dip the tip of their right ring finger in the clay, then place the palm of their right hand on their forehead and drag that same ring finger up the bridge of their nose, passing the third eye to the base of their palm, making two straight vertical lines while chanting the mantra *om keshavaya namaha*. They were like fine artists. I didn't know it at the time, but the monks also applied it to different parts of their bodies—belly, chest, throat, the sides of the abdomen, above the elbows, shoulders, lower back, upper back, and the top of the head, where only a tuft of hair remains—while chanting other mantras. Hindu monks shave their head, except for a tuft of hair called a shikha, which is kept in a ponytail on the crown of the head. It's over the thousand-petaled lotus chakra. The shikha is said to fine-tune intelligence and energize spiritual centers. In Ayurveda the shikha protects a point on the head known as the adhipati marma (or meridian) and is said to be the nexus of all nerves. In yogic anatomy the subtle energy channel known as the shushumna rises from the lower chakras to a part of the brain called the brahma randhra. It's right above that brahma randhra that the shikha rests on the head.

The monks basically ignored me. Not in a bad way—it was as if they were on a mission from God and paid no attention to me. I was just some kid in surf shorts. One monk was slower than the rest. He was a young guy around my age. Green. New to this, I guessed, but trying earnestly.

"What's your name, Prabhu?" *Prabhu* was a kind way of addressing somebody, anybody, as *master.*

"Ray," I answered.

"Bhakta Ray, my name's Bhakta Jason." In the ashram they added *bhakta* before every name, which meant "devoted" or "devotee." It was also a sign that a person had not taken on a spiritual initiation, after which *das,* meaning "servant," was added at the end of the name. Bada Hari would formally be addressed as Bada Hari Das. Usually, the monk's new name was a name of God.

"What are you doing?" Bhakta Jason asked. "Mangala arati"—the early morning temple program—"is about to start. You've only got five minutes to get there, and you didn't even shower yet."

"I figure I'm going to the beach later today," I said.

"You can't go into the temple to see the Lord unshowered, Bhakta Ray!" he said. "You don't want to present yourself like that. Saucham, external cleanliness, is important. And when you wake up you should immediately start chanting the *Mahamantra*," he said. This is your internal saucham."

I didn't mind his rebuke. I supposed he probably got corrected as a junior monk and was now passing it on to me. I wanted to learn anyway. He insisted I had to take a shower before I went to the temple, so I acquiesced. He was late to rise, anyway, so I think I served as a good scapegoat for him being late to the temple program.

"How long have you been into this, Jason?" I asked. He looked like a California surfer with a long, blond tuft of hair.

"I got a book when I was twelve years old in Albany, New York," he said. "I read it cover to cover, and I felt like this one book had all the answers to life. As early as I could, I took off to India and went on a pilgrimage to the holy places."

I was surprised and inspired. He looked a bit younger than me, but he already had more spiritual depth and experience.

In the shower, I noticed there was no handle on the hot water, making cold the only option. I went quickly, dried off, and there was Jason, waiting for me.

"Ray, you've given thousands of lives to maya," he said, referring to the Vedic concept of illusion. "Why not give just this one short life to Krishna?" He spoke with conviction, but it lacked the depth a seasoned practitioner had.

"How do you know there's not just one life?" I asked.

He said nothing, but looked at me as if I was a helpless doubter. I wasn't. But I wasn't convinced.

* * *

In the temple, while the other monks chanted I stood in awe of the paintings that Zack and I had looked at the day before. It was a scheduled quiet chanting time, which happened between about 5:30 and 7:30 a.m. I walked around with some mala beads loaned to me by Bada Hari, but I was distracted by all the beautiful paintings.

Bada Hari saw me staring at one of them. I looked at him, breaking the silence, and whispered, "What's going on in this painting?"

"This is the Kirtan Avatar, the great master Lord Chaitanya, and he's carrying the body of Haridas, who just died."

"Who's Haridas?" I asked.

"This was from a time when India was ruled by Muslims. They wreaked terror in Hindu communities, slaughtered literally hundreds of thousands. They became especially disturbed if one of their own became attracted to bhakti, or the yoga of devotion. Haridas was born into a Muslim family, but he understood that Vedic thought is inclusive. It teaches that there is one God and that when you really love God, you'll see God in every being. The concept of 'us and them' and 'my religion versus your religion' is a moot point in Vedic thought. We are all spirit souls, but we've just forgotten. The goal of religion is to help us remember that we're all connected. You'll understand different spiritual paths as different ways to approach God. You won't see other paths as rivals; you'll see them as kindred spirits. So Haridas understood this. He understood the connection between all of us, and he dove deep into these teachings. The fanatical rulers were furious and merely saw him as a heretic. He would simply state Vedic teachings. 'We are all spiritual beings. God is one. Treat everyone with dignity and love.' Fanatics cannot hear this."

"There are fanatics in every tradition," I said. "I've encountered them."

"Yes, Ray, but the truth is the truth. No one person, religion, or country owns the truth. Truth is food for the spirit. Haridas understood this, so they threatened to imprison him unless he gave up what they called Hindu rituals. He argued that chanting the *Mahamantra* is not a Hindu ritual; it is the soul calling for God. That desire to reconnect with God is inherent in all traditions."

"They're just different names for the same God," I clarified.

"Yes. To call it a Hindu ritual is to limit it to a geographic or bodily designation. The soul wants to call out to God, and Vedic culture teaches us how to do it. So, he continued and told the fanatics, 'No, I cannot give this up. This gives me so much joy and makes me feel so connected. Why would I ever give it up?' They threatened him with prison. 'If you must, put me in prison,' he said. But when people are spiritually connected, even prison cannot bother them. Understand this, Ray, if you do this process correctly, there is no prison that can ever hold you. You start to realize that the only real prison is your own mind and senses, which have the ability to bind you. The great yogis want freedom, but not in a political or social way. That is secondary. Real freedom means controlling your mind and senses."

I felt like I was getting a massive truth bomb, and I smiled. I could still hear the hum of the other monks chanting softly on their beads as I stood, captivated by conversation, with our bare feet on the cool temple floor.

"When people are focused on their spiritual life, nothing can hurt them," he said. "Inspired living inspires other people. That's exactly what happened. In that prison cell, he inspired all the prisoners to start chanting the *Mahamantra*."

"You're kidding," I said. "His captors must have hated that."

"They did. They were furious. They considered it insubordination. But we would call it his fixation on truth and love. He was ordered to be publicly beaten in twenty-two marketplaces and finally put to death."

"Horrific," I mumbled, eyes widened. "The public beatings were to set an example?"

"Exactly. This is how invaders often ruled. But something strange happened, Ray. Haridas was so not of this world, so enraptured by the love of the soul and of God, that they could not hurt him. Even though he was lashed and beaten, his face was joyful. He couldn't be a victim. He understood that they were merely hurting his body, and they couldn't touch him."

"This must have infuriated his enemies even more."

"It did. And after the twenty-second marketplace where Haridas didn't respond—didn't even seem disturbed—they thought, *Maybe this guy is a saint. Maybe he is a mystic. Maybe he is a Hindu god of sorts.* Those cruel guards who were beating him relentlessly looked at him, puzzled, and broke down. 'We're sorry. We've been ordered to kill you, but nothing we do is even bothering you. We feel as if we've enacted a crime against you. You must be some great soul. But if we don't kill you, they will kill us.'

"Haridas was shocked and saddened. 'They will kill you?' he said compassionately to his perpetrators. With all the love in his heart, he was broken that these people, the very people that were trying to kill him, would be killed by their superiors. He said, 'I don't want them to kill you. I'm sorry I have not died. I will die immediately.' Haridas sat in a mystical trance and, using yogic siddhis, halted all apparent life in his material body."

"I've heard that's a siddhi some yogis can perform!"

"Yes! He did it, and he seemed to be dead, although he was merely in a state of suspended animation. Then the guards threw his body in the Ganges River. Haridas, still alive, woke from his trance and swam downstream, where he met the other devotees."

"That's an amazing story," I said. "It's like Jesus praying for the people that nailed him to the cross. 'Father, forgive them, for they know not what they are doing.'"

"Exactly. A great master sees that even those acting in cruel ways are merely covered by illusion, and therefore they do not hate them. They pray for them and wish them well and pray for spiritual connection themselves. If you're on this path, Ray, you cannot ever let hateful people make you hate. If you do, then hate wins."

* * *

My stay at the Krishna temple in Laguna Beach gave me some insight into the bhakti path. When I returned to New York, I decided to learn more from the local Krishnas. They had a bigger ashram in downtown Brooklyn than the one I'd been to on Greenwich Avenue, so I decided to go there. Brooklyn was scary. Our street on North Eighth was the only safe one at this point in the 1980s, and I didn't venture out too much. But I was eager to check out this ashram, so I rolled the dice with my safety.

That subway stop was in a dangerous area of Atlantic Avenue. Sometimes, a handful of us would go to the ashram for a Sunday lecture and feast because there was safety in numbers. The temple there was big and slightly intimidating. I was struggling philosophically with the idea that came up a lot in yoga that God was an energy. An amorphous power. A light. A positive, loving force. I'd heard this described in many of the yoga books of Ramana Maharshi. I had gone through a period of diving into the Upanishads and Christian theologians such as Thomas Aquinas and Bede Griffiths, who spoke of God as a force or a "higher power," a formless or divine entity. It didn't necessarily sit well with me, but I was open to the idea. The more I studied different traditions, the more I realized the two paradigms of truth (God is formless or God has form) were in constant conflict. I strongly desired to understand this and get to the bottom of it.

This temple in Brooklyn was crowded and culturally diverse. Everyone seemed to know what they were doing, and I felt like an outsider. I didn't really know anyone. I just wandered around the temple, which had a gift shop near the front desk. There was a corridor before you went into the massive temple room. The corridor was cool because it had retro black-and-white photos on the wall of A. C. Bhaktivedanta Swami when he first came to New York City in the 1960s and '70s. They depicted Western converts and their swami draped in Indian garb on the Lower East Side, walking the same streets I walked.

The temple itself was a little overwhelming. The kirtan was different from anywhere else I'd been. Usually, the call-and-response chanting was gentle, peaceful, and frankly, a little boring for my taste at the various yoga centers I'd been to. This was not. This was hordes of people jumping up and down, some with drums strapped around their bodies. Five drummers played as tightly as a marching band. The lower drumhead thumped like a sonic boom as each drummer pounded on the skins exactly at the same time. It was tribal. It was big. Many deftly played karatalas, ranging in size from a silver dollar to a dinner plate. They sizzled like the hi-hat of a drum set. The singer, a Black man with a beautiful voice, led the group in call-and-response and free-form dancing up and down the temple floor like a parade. He brought the chanting up to a high-speed tempo and then dropped it off a cliff to a slow, almost dragging beat. Adults were hopping, as if outside of their bodies, feeling a pleasure shown through their smiles, screaming, and singing the response of the mantra. The joy on their faces was contagious, and I couldn't help but smile.

The altar was two marble statues of deities, which I later found out were Krishna and Radha, as the devotees worship God as both male and female. I loved the concept that for God to be whole, both masculine and feminine must be present. The deities were dressed in wild, magnificent outfits with sequins and bright, gaudy colors. They were garlanded with beautiful roses and wore gold and silver crowns, ornaments, jewelry, and ankle bells, making the entire visual seem almost extravagant. A simple priest wore white draped cloth, and instead of a shirt, another white cloth covered half his chest. He rang bells and waved five incense sticks clockwise around the deities. He did it in a graceful way, in massive circles with artistic wrist movements, which made it seem like part of a beautiful performance. But he wasn't facing the audience. He was facing the deities, looking at them lovingly, as if they were looking back into his eyes.

Conch shells were blown. Brass oil lamps were waved in circles at the statues and then handed to a person in the audience to walk around the crowd. The crowd magnetically moved toward the fiery lamp, placing their hands above the flames, close enough to feel the heat but not close enough to get burned, and then touched their warm hands to their foreheads. Some people threw dollar bills on the plate that the lamp was on. What a way to gather donations!

The temple must have been a former synagogue or Masonic temple. It was basically empty with a wood floor, three- or four-story-high ceilings, and a balcony. Like the Laguna Beach temple, beautiful paintings of Hindu gods and goddesses lined the walls. In the center of the floor, toward the back and facing the altar, was a statue of the guru sitting on a raised cushion chair. The statue was so lifelike I did a double take—it could have been a man in deep meditation.

As I walked out the back door of the temple to the front lobby, there were tables covered in books and snacks. Spicy pakoras, samosas, and Indian sweets. Hundreds of books piqued my interest: *The Perfection of Yoga, Beyond Birth and Death*, and *The Nectar of Devotion* to name a few. Then I came upon a book I already owned, one of my favorite books at the time: *Food for the Spirit: Vegetarianism and the World Religions*, by Steven Rosen. It presented how prominent world religions all supported a restricted diet when it came to animal consumption. It was filled with facts, quotes, and scriptural references that I used when endorsing animal rights among religious people who consumed meat.

I wondered if the author was part of this sect of the Krishna community or if the ashram just carried his book. Then I noticed a tall man standing close, peering over my shoulder. He was dressed conventionally, in a blazer and jeans. I immediately recognized his smile from the back of *Food for the Spirit.*

"Oh, hi!" I said. "You're the author! I use your book constantly. I'm a vegetarian and animal rights supporter. Your book is a fantastic resource! I'm so honored and excited to meet you. Are you a Krishna, too?"

"Yes, definitely," he replied.

"You don't look like one by the way you're dressed," I said.

"Our spiritual life has little to do with the way we dress, and more to do with what's in our head and heart. Wouldn't you agree?"

Good answer! I thought, and nodded.

"I'm going to buy *Food for the Spirit* for my friend Maryanne. Can I ask you a spiritual question about Vedic teachings?"

"Sure."

"There seems to be a discrepancy in different traditions. Some worship God as a personal deity and some as formless. It seems reckless to dive into a tradition before getting to the bottom of this. What does the Vedic tradition say about personal or impersonal facets of God?"

"There are both," he replied simply.

"How could God be both? Isn't God either one or the other?"

"Is the sun different from the sun's rays?"

"Yes," I said. Then I caught myself. "Well, yes and no."

"Which is it?" he poked. "Can you separate them from each other?"

"I guess you can't have one without the other, but in one sense they are different. Like if I say the sun is in the room, I'm not talking about the planet, I'm—"

"Yes, exactly," he said. "They are different, and they are one. One is the sun globe, and one is the energy of the sun. Neither are wrong, but it's looking at Truth, God, or our Higher Power from different vantage points. If I'm looking at a drawing of a number 9 written on a piece of paper, my intelligence accepts it as a 9. A person across from me sees the same drawing, but from his perspective, it's a 6. We're seeing the same thing from different vantage points. Only fools would say, 'I see a 6, and you are wrong,' or, 'I see a 9, and *you* are wrong!'

"This misunderstanding of truth through different vantage points has destroyed spiritual traditions throughout the world. It must be uprooted."

I had to agree. And since he was being deeply philosophical, I thought I'd throw some other questions at him. "I've run into a lot of people that say truth is subjective," I said. "That *their* truth might be different from my truth. They say that truth is in the mind of the beholder and that there's no such thing as absolute truth."

"So they say without doubt that truth is subjective?" he asked, smiling. "That, Ray, is an absolute statement."

We both laughed.

"God, that makes so much sense," I said.

"Look, Ray, you seem bright. People who argue that we all have our own truth are fooling themselves. They cannot live with good conscience. That's like saying 'Adolf Hitler had his truth. Let him do what he wants. Pol Pot, Mussolini, Stalin had their own truths. Let them be. It's *their* truth.' No. This makes no sense whatsoever. There *is* truth, and there *is* illusion. There *is* love, and there *is* hate. There *is* light, and there *is* darkness."

I nodded. He was right. There had to be a gold standard of truth for all people, all seekers, that was not bound by nation, culture, or religion.

"People also argue there is no right or wrong."

"Do you believe that?" he asked.

"No," I said. "There must be."

"People are fools," he said. "They'll say anything to justify doing whatever the hell they want to do. Of course there's a right and wrong. Or are they saying that kidnapping and human trafficking are okay?" He smiled at how ridiculous people could be in the name of deep philosophical thinking. "Good luck living *that* reality."

I had to smile as well. Because he answered clearly and concisely, I asked him more of my deep questions.

"There's another group of people who argue that the body is a machine, there is no God, no spirit, no truth, and we are just matter that will rot into the earth when we die," I said. "Religion was created to control us. We should be free to live to our highest amount of ecstasy, but we repress it because of some social doctrine that makes us repress our inherent joy. If we were really free, we would break down all these formal ideas of marriage and social structures and engage freely in sense indulgence, where we could live out our sexual freedom, unrestricted by the formal, archaic rituals. We're no different from animals, but we've artificially created restrictions that we follow from our predecessors, and it's crippled our society and cheated us out of deep inherent joy."

He nodded. "Yes, people speak like this naively," he said. "Where have you ever found indulgence giving one joy, Ray? It may give you excitement. It may give you a thrill, but you'd be naive if you think indulgence of the senses gives you joy. Talk to anyone in rehab or a twelve-step program about the so-called joys of indulgence. See where it got them. After speaking to them, you'll get a much more accurate picture of indulgence and its results."

"But what about sexual repression?" I asked desperately. "Didn't Freud say it manifests in horrible ways?"

"Yes, you don't subjugate or repress it. You sublimate it. Transform. Transmute it. Purify it to something much higher."

I immediately loved this man and asked if he came to this temple regularly.

"Yes, every morning at 7 a.m. I live around the corner."

"Can I come and ask you more questions if I come at 7 a.m.?"

He smiled and nodded his head.

"You're Steven? Or Mr. Rosen?" I asked.

"Since we have a spiritual relationship, you can call me the name my guru gave me—Satyaraja Das."

*　　*　　*

I decided to go to the Brooklyn temple every morning at 7 a.m. for kirtan and class on the *Srimad Bhagavatam*, one of the ancient Hindu literatures, since I knew Satyaraja Das would be there as he promised.

After kirtan and the class, I went downstairs into a large, dark, finished basement. All the temple residents sat on the floor. We were served breakfast on metal plates like you'd imagine in a mess hall in the army. I sat next to Satyaraja as they served delicious kitchari (lentils cooked with rice, turmeric, chilis, and other spices) with tomato chutney and papadams (thin crackers made with lentil flour and chunks of peppercorns, which occasionally made me cough). It was a simple but healthy breakfast, and it was their staple in the ashram. Two men would come around and humbly serve piping hot chapatis, like puffed tortillas, covered in ghee.

Satyaraja ate fastidiously, and I dove right into my morning questions. I came every day, and every day his answers were sound, rooted in tradition, practicality, and above all common sense. I felt like he was the one person that spoke my language and that God and the universe had sent him to me. I really had a heart connection with this man. I didn't feel like he wanted anything from me. Because he dressed conventionally and scholarly, I could relate to him. It didn't freak me out at all. He was approachable, kind, and funny. He had a deep mental sobriety that seemed much more grounded than Guru James, from the nightclub, who seemed slightly more pretentious and more frivolous in his God-realization. After my experience with the mushrooms he gave me, I found out Guru James was having sex with one of the girls from the nightclub, and I lost faith in him. Frivolous promiscuity didn't seem like an act of the self-realized. I had also started to notice that he'd randomly take things from different traditions, if not downright make up things. Guru James resembled a charismatic, self-proclaimed guru posing as a spiritual leader, but he did not align with any spiritual tradition and did not, apparently, adhere to ethical behavior. On the other hand, there was nothing pretentious about Satyaraja. He was grave, deep, yet fun and relatable, like a friend or wise uncle. And every now and then, he'd just shut me down. With a smile.

"Satyaraja, I've been told by a teacher that I am God and some mantras will help me remember it," I said, thinking about what Guru James had once told me.

"If you're God, how did you fall into illusion?"

*   *   *

My conversations with Satyaraja Das were always straightforward, deep, and focused, which is why he caught me off guard one morning when he asked an apparently frivolous question: "What kind of guitar does your guitar player use?"

We never spoke of anything but deep spiritual questions and answers, so I didn't understand why he asked such an out-of-character question. "He plays a Gibson Les Paul," I said. "Why do you ask?"

"Oh, because I used to play guitar and loved it, but I gave it up."

"You gave it up?" I asked, surprised. "Why?"

He shrugged his shoulders meekly and said, "For me, it was maya," referring to the illusory energy of the world.

I was confused. "But you told me and you taught me that everything we have in this world is a gift from God and we should use it in God's service."

He shrugged his shoulders. "Yes, but for me it was maya."

That answer just wasn't good enough for me. "But you told me the *Bhagavad Gita* recommends taking what we have and using it in a way to purify ourselves instead of degrading ourselves. You told me, utility is the principle. That something like music isn't good or bad; it's how it's used. You used the example of a knife. You said a knife could be used to slit a throat or save someone's life in a delicate operation. It's all in how it's used, Satyaraja. Why would you give it up after instructing me like this?" I was getting worked up. Why wasn't he teaching me the entire truth, or why was he not following his truth? My eyes bulged when he repeated the same thing.

"That is all true, but for me it was just too much. It was maya."

Unhappy and dissatisfied, I pushed him more. "But you always encourage me to do music. You've said that I can do it as an offering. I cannot understand why you're taking this position now. I say this in all humility, but truthfully I'm a little shocked."

He got very serious and looked me in the eye. "Okay, Ray, next time you're on stage, see if you're doing it to *serve* God or to *be* God!"

My jaw dropped. This was a paradigm shift. It spun my brain around. I knew right then without having to get on stage that my entire performance on stage was to *be* God. Be the center. A mad search for validation. It wasn't about serving; it was about me. With all my so-called altruism, clean living, self-betterment, my deeper motivation was to stake my claim for self-importance, and this realization was a death blow to my material agenda.

Satyaraja's question stayed with me. It changed the way I performed on stage. It changed the way I lived in the present moment. It changed how I taught and how I related to my family. *Am I here to serve God or be God?* I realized that, yes, everything we had could be used for God, but at the same time, a wise person may voluntarily give something up if they felt like it was too overwhelming for the ego. Satyaraja's renunciation wasn't false; it was due to deep understanding of his own limitations with his ego and his sincerity on his path.

On the spiritual path, there were people, places, and things that could deeply trigger us. They pushed buttons. They were the slippery slopes that took us downhill fast. It was not evil to have triggers, but triggers were danger zones to be respected for the disaster they could cause.

*　　*　　*

Because I had lost faith in Guru James, I quit the nightclub job. It wasn't the magic mushrooms, either. Finding out that he was having sex with employees ruined his integrity for me, but the last straw was the night he invited me to a spiritual gathering at his luxurious home on the Upper West Side. Maryanne and many others from the club were also invited.

He had a beautiful townhouse that was decorated in a medieval-meets-new-age style. Gigantic paintings of angels hung on the wall, and a suit of armor holding a battle-axe stood in the doorway. The biggest purple amethyst I had ever seen sparkled, spotlighted from below. There was a zebra-skin rug on the floor of the entry, which was beautiful but grossed me out. The walls were wooden, and I noticed an impressive collection of occult books on the built-in oak shelves. He had a few elegant crystal chandeliers, their lights dimmed, while frankincense pleasantly choked me. About fifteen of us sat in a circle on cushions while a servant brought us jasmine tea. We meditated quietly for about twenty minutes before Guru James burst into the room, as dramatic as ever, wearing a purple velvet robe and carrying a sword.

Oh my God, this guy is nuts, I thought.

By the time he led us through an abundance mantra, or chanting for money, I had had enough of it. I took Maryanne aside and explained my lack of faith in Guru James. "He seems like a wealthy spiritual charlatan," I said. "Perhaps not evil; I just think he's deluded. I don't buy it anymore."

Maryanne nodded. "The chanting for money thing threw me off, too," she said. "It seems like when there's faith in God, money mantras are ridiculous."

I agreed. There couldn't be more of a contrast between Guru James and Satyaraja, who I respected more and more each day. The next time I saw him at the temple, we ate kitchari and papadams together as usual.

"It's the most warming and grounding food I've ever eaten," I said.

". . . and cooked with love," he added.

"Satyaraja, what do you think of magic mushrooms?" I asked, thinking about Guru James.

"What do *you* think of them?"

"It seems they can be tools for higher consciousness," I said. "I never would have done them, but a teacher recommended them to me. I took them and . . . well, my loudest realization was that everything I had ever read in the *Bhagavad Gita* was true. In one sense they gave me faith in the teachings of the Vedas. So, I'm grateful for them."

Satyaraja looked at me and nodded soberly. "Yes, they can do that. But at the same time, people can also take them and have the opposite experience. We've all heard of bad trips. Not every trip is the same. Right?"

I nodded.

"Your experience was real. Your message was profound. But don't mistake the flute for the player of the flute, Ray," he said. "Krishna was behind the message, not the mushrooms."

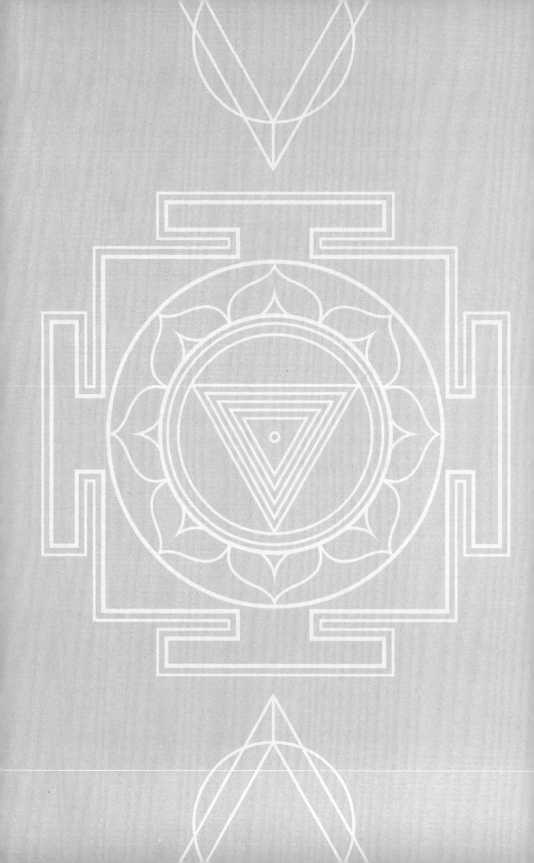

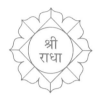

CHAPTER 6

BECOMING A BRAHMACHARI

Youth of Today got offered a record deal from Caroline Records. Up to that point, we had released all our own records on our own label. We did everything ourselves for the most part. Now, a bigger independent record company was offering to put out our new record for us and give us a monetary advance on royalties. We were shocked. This label had put out bands like White Zombie and the Misfits, and now they wanted to sign us.

In those days (and even today), most bands didn't make any money. In fact, they usually paid to play. By the time you tallied up all the costs for equipment, rehearsal space, renting or buying a van, and everything else, most bands were financially underwater. Youth of Today never had any money either, so when Caroline Records offered us $25,000 for our new LP, it might as well have been $25 million.

Of course, with money came a bunch of interpersonal wars about dividing up the money that never existed when we were broke: *I wrote all the songs; I should get more. I booked the shows; I should get something for that! I've been paying for all this equipment that's been money out of my pocket the band never paid for; I need to get reimbursed for that.*

It's amazing how success can complicate life.

After accepting the deal, we got more press and interviews in magazines, fanzines, and even *Night Flight*, one of the first video music shows that pre-dated MTV. This drew new fans, random haters, and hatred from some people we thought were close to us. Loyal fans became envious of our good fortune, and it hurt me to the core of my being.

But the lyrics on the record, *We're Not in This Alone*, reflected my spir-itual inspiration. We also had one final lineup change that really clicked. We had a new drummer, fifteen-year-old Sammy Siegler, and a new bass-ist, seventeen-year-old Walter Schreifels from Queens, who played in a small local band called Gorilla Biscuits, which I had signed to Revelation Records. Decades later Sammy and Walter went on to play in huge bands that toured the world many times over, and Gorilla Biscuits became one of the biggest hardcore bands of all time.

But at that moment, we had booked our biggest US tour to date, and things appeared more promising than ever. At the same time, I was getting pulled in a different direction. I knew we were doing a good thing. I knew our message was positive and changing people's lives. Unfortunately, I felt I wasn't growing as a person, and it was killing me. I was a little more famous now. Big deal! I had more people at each performance we played. Big deal! I made a little bit more money. Big deal! More girls (and guys) thought I was cooler. Big deal! Nothing excited me. I felt stagnant. Amid all the thrill, I wanted out.

I had a burning desire to go to India and find myself. I wanted to detox from the world of hardcore music. I wanted to follow the path of the sages that I read about in books. There was nothing here for me anymore. No amount of money, no sexual intimacy, no number of fans could give me what my soul really yearned for. Any fame I got with the band was not making me a better person; it was merely amplifying my ego and my entitlement, which in turn made me more distressed.

Underneath all this excitement was my father's condition. He had been in a coma now for almost three years, the entire time I had been in New York, and it was eating away at me no matter how much I stuck my head in the sand. Seeing my mother go through her distressed yet loyal devotion to him, a situation that was completely out of her control, gave me a deep sadness and lack of faith in the material world. It painted an accurate, bleak picture of existence—no matter how solid life appears, it was nothing more than a sandcastle when the waves of time and fate came to shore. Nobody got a pass from tragedy, trauma, or reversals in life. This was everyone's destiny.

My God calling was getting louder and louder each day. After my meeting Satyaraja and studying the *Bhagavad Gita*, my direction in bhakti yoga came into clearer focus. Considering all of this, I couldn't figure out why God was sending me on the tour. I loved the guys in the band. They were like my brothers, but they were kids in my eyes, and in their eyes I was losing my mind. They didn't get me, and that was going to make traveling confined in a van together difficult. Every instinct told me I was ripe to leave all of this behind. It seemed like the natural flow of things, although I knew the band would be let down.

Four days before the tour, the used van we'd bought broke down beyond repair. Our long-term roadie had quit the tour, and I thought this might be a whisper from the universe to change course. Then, one day later, Steve Reddy, our old friend, fan, and show promoter of Youth of Today in Albany, New York, reached out to me. "I heard your van broke down and you need a roadie," he said. "I've got nothing to do this summer, and I have a van. I'll road manage you guys and take you on tour if you like."

At that moment, I realized that God had sent me a kindred spirit for the tour. Steve was a year older than me, responsible, mature, and sick of the material world. We connected on a deep level and created a bond on that tour that accelerated our spiritual journeys. We read together, distributed cases of the *Bhagavad Gita* at our merch table, and even visited ashrams along the way. By the time we made it back to New York City three months later, we were ready for a God quest and materially exhausted. That coincidentally happened to be the holy day of Krishna Janmashtami, Krishna's birthday, and the day we both chose to give our life to our spiritual calling.

I told my band that I loved them but I was quitting and not sure if I'd ever play again. They were all a little shocked, perhaps hurt and confused. We had just finished out biggest tour, and it seemed like we were on the brink of getting even bigger. It seemed like I was throwing away all that we had worked for. But I was convinced that there was nothing of this material world that would satisfy my heart. I wanted God. Spirit. Higher love. Krishna. I wanted what sages from cultures around the globe had received, giving up the temporary for the eternal. I wanted what mystics and saints embraced, and I wanted to walk away from what they walked away from. I was bored with maya, and I didn't want escapism through drugs, romance, or busyness. I knew it was time to move on.

When I called home to my mother to tell her my plans, I found out my father, after three years in a coma, had just died.

*   *   *

I put on a suit for the first time since high school. My entire family was there for my father's wake in Connecticut. It was surreal to see my father in the casket. Lying stiff. In makeup. Like a mannequin. So peculiar. He lay there, uncommonly thin. It was tough for me to witness. It was so unlike his robust Italian, pasta-eating body that I was used to, that I held, embraced, smelled. But it was him. Or at least his body. And I cried, having never lost anything or anyone of this value. A person that would love me unconditionally. It was also a cry of relief, knowing what my mother had been through for the past three years.

Some people see a person in a coma as a patient, mute and paralyzed, while others see the living dead. I dealt with my father's ambiguous state by not dealing with it. I never knew what to say to him or whether what I was saying was heard. I shut off my feelings completely, with an occasional outburst of tears. The coma didn't go away though. My father's body got thinner, his face gaunter. I went on with my life, leaving my mother to deal with it. I was shamefully checked out for three years. Numb. Unable to process. Or merely self-absorbed, typical for a teenager. Checked into my band, my music, my scene. But regardless, it was shameful and humiliating in retrospect.

This dark chapter was illumined only by the sense that it drove me to search for shelter beyond the material world. The mantra "there is no safety here" ran through the back of my mind. At any moment, the material world can pull the carpet out from beneath your feet, snuffing out dreams and fantastic plans.

At the wake, I stood in line behind family and relatives to say goodbye and take a final view of the body. The soul is eternal; the body is a shell. This truth helped me frame the loss. I covertly held a small vial of water from the Ganges River, which a monk at the ashram had given me. "It helps release the spirit to move forward," the monk had said. I poured it in my hand and clandestinely sprinkled the sacred liquid on his body.

After the goodbyes, tears, and solemn embraces, I walked down to the corner market to get two passport photos. Dad passed away on a holy day, the day commemorating Krishna's birth. Many of the monks in the ashram in Brooklyn told me this was a very auspicious time for his soul to leave. That helped me cope with the loss to a degree. For weeks, and even months, after, I had recurring dreams of my father as I remembered him—but dressed in the saffron robes of a renunciate. He would see me in my neophyte stage as a practitioner and encourage me on my spiritual path.

My father left. Now I had to leave. I soon received my passport. Steve Reddy had moved to a Krishna farm in rural Pennsylvania to become a monk farmer. I wrote to a guesthouse in Vrindavan, a holy town in northern India, asked if I could stay there, and said that I would follow any principles the monks followed. I wanted to practice brahmacharya—the act of giving up the pleasures of the five senses (including sex) in pursuit of spiritual liberation and sacred knowledge. Students of brahmacharya are called brahmacharis, and they live a strict, simple lifestyle in the ashram with others on the spiritual path, including elder monks who can guide you. It usually involves chanting and meditation, restricting the diet to sacred foods, studying wisdom texts, and practicing cleanliness and nonviolence.

When I received the piece of ultralight airmail from Vrindavan confirming my reservation, I booked an open-ended ticket from JFK to the airport in Delhi.

* * *

I had always had a desire to go to England. It was a material desire, but I figured I may as well lay over there and visit the Krishna temple on Soho Street in London. That's how I justified it. I walked in the door and told them I was on my way to India to search for God, and they allowed me to stay on the ashram floor with the other monks for four days. I enjoyed menial service in their kitchen, washing pots and sweeping up.

This was one of the Western cities where the Krishna teachings were spread so vigorously by George Harrison and the Beatles. I wondered if I would see George. (I found out later that he and I were in India at the same time.) I sat in the temple room alone, quietly chanting on my mala beads, attempting to be meditative and focused. But I was distracted, curious, and unsettled. I picked up a songbook and opened it to a random page. I read a Bengali poem translated into English:

> The spiritual master is receiving benedictions from
> the ocean of mercy. Just as a rain cloud extinguishes
> a forest fire, the spiritual master extinguishes the
> blazing forest fire of material existence. I offer my
> respectful obeisances to the lotus feet of such a spiri-
> tual master, who is an ocean of auspicious qualities.

That is the most beautiful thing I've ever read! I thought. *This material world* is *like a blazing forest fire!* I copied the quotation down in my diary so I wouldn't forget it. Just then, a sweet young couple, about twenty-nine years old, came and introduced themselves to me as Maria and Jonathan. I shared the verse with them.

"Yes, when a forest fire takes over, they call so many fire departments to put them out," said Jonathan in a charming English accent. "Even planes and helicopters. But often it's a futile effort. But, sometimes, by good fortune, it begins to rain. Only that rain cloud has the ability to destroy the fire. Our teachers come to us almost magically and offer us knowledge, truth, values, and information to assist us in escaping this blazing fire of the material world. This material world can get quite hot. You think so, Ray?"

"Yes! For sure!" I nodded. "I've been burned by the material world in that very fire, but I've also felt some relief in reading the sacred literature. I feel like it sheds light on the confusing aspects of life."

They took me around London, treating me like a younger brother. Their kindness and their sweet, soft natures won my heart. Jonathan could eloquently explain the philosophy of the *Gita*. They returned me to the temple room where they'd found me and went on their way. I sat back down and started flicking through more songbooks. Then a familiar face, dressed casually but funky, came into the temple, bowed down, and chanted on beads. I tried not to be obvious, but the fanboy in me kicked in. It was Poly Styrene, the singer of one of my favorite bands, X-Ray Spex. They were one of the original punk bands of the late 1970s in England, pioneers of the genre that took the world by storm. They rubbed elbows with the Buzzcocks, the Sex Pistols, and the Clash. They knew everyone who was anyone. But X-Ray Spex? They were my favorite. I had all their singles and all the posters of them on my wall in my teen years. I heard that Poly Styrene had become a devotee of Krishna, and now she was sitting ten feet from me in a lotus position chanting softly on beads. I didn't say anything.

This is stupid, I thought. *I should just go up and tell her I appreciate her work. Does that sound dumb? Fans did it to me all the time.* I was paralyzed. After twenty minutes, she got up to leave, and I darted toward her.

"Hi, you don't know me but . . . I'll say it," I said. "I'm your biggest fan. Love you. You are Poly Styrene, right?"

She smiled sweetly. "Yes. What's your name?"

"Ray. I'm in a band," I said. "I mean . . . I was in a band. Do I sound like a quitter? Maybe I shouldn't have said that. What I mean to say is that I'm on a search for God."

"Well, Ray," she said, "I'm walking down to the studio to record some music. Would you like to walk with me?"

"Yes!" I said loudly by mistake, losing my cool. We got our jackets on and headed for the recording studio.

"Are you into all this Krishna stuff?" I asked sincerely as we walked side by side.

"Yes, of course!" she said. "My spiritual name is Maharani. It's a name for Krishna's consort Radha. What was your band like? Why did you quit? Was it too much maya?"

"Truthfully the guys in the band are cool," I said. "We were all into punk and hardcore. We all loved your band. It just was maya for me."

"Did you sing about drugs or partying or politics?" she asked.

"No, we actually sang about *not* doing drugs and becoming vegetarians."

"That sounds great!" She lit up. "Did anybody become vegetarians because of it?"

"Yeah!" I said. "Like thousands of people . . . but they did not become spiritualists."

We continued walking for about ten minutes, then stood outside of her studio.

"If you can turn thousands of people into vegetarians with good lyrics, music, and intelligence, you may one day be able to end a world war!" she said.

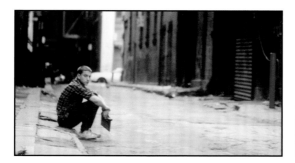
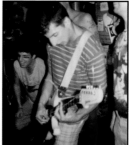
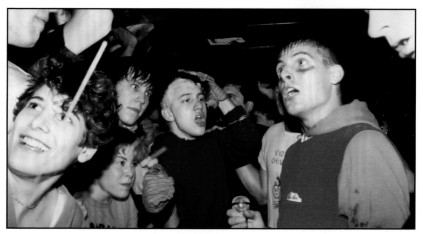
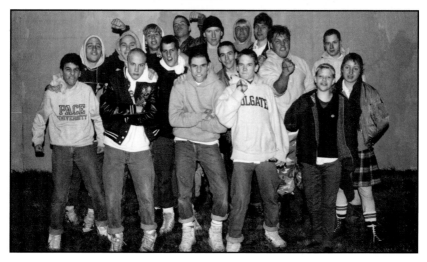

TOP LEFT: Ray in Greenwich Village, NYC, 1981. Photo by Thomas Cappo. TOP RIGHT: Porcell and Kevin Seconds at the Anthrax, Stamford, CT, 1984. Photo by Jamie Keever. MIDDLE: Ray and crowd sing along with 7 Seconds at the Anthrax, Stamford, CT, 1984. Photo by Jamie Keever. BOTTOM: Youth crew at the Anthrax, Stamford, CT, 1986. Photo by Chris Schneider.

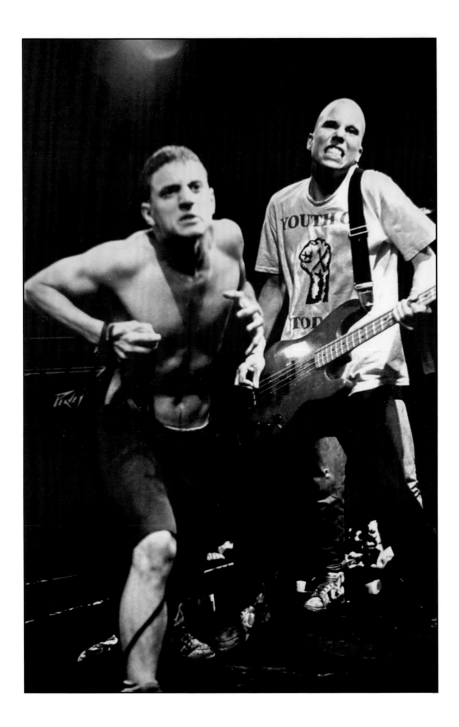

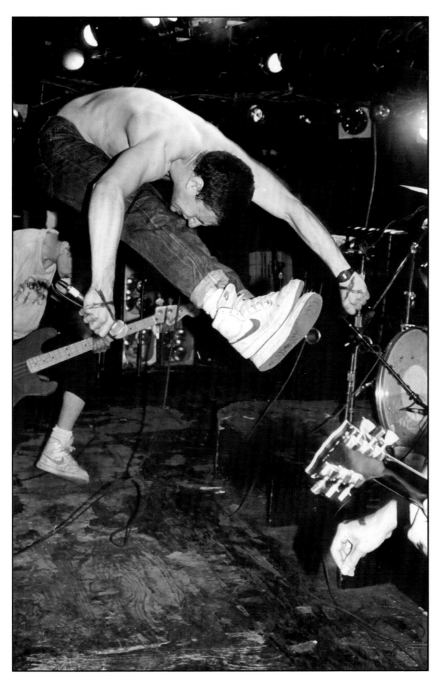

OPPOSITE: Youth of Today with Craig Ahead from Sick of It All on bass at CBGB, NYC, 1986. Photo by Bri Hurley. ABOVE: Youth of Today at the Rathskellar, Boston, MA, 1986. Photo by JJ Gonson.

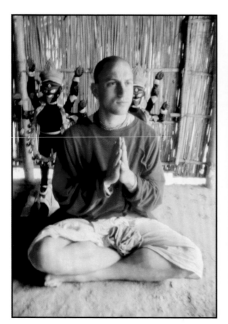
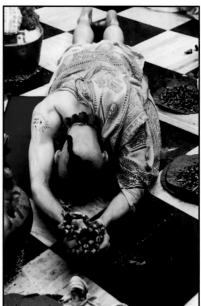
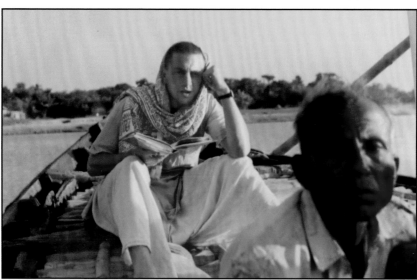

TOP LEFT: Ray at Kali Puja in Nabadwip, West Bengal, India, 1988. TOP RIGHT: Ray receiving the name "Raghunath" and his japa mala in Vrindavan, Uttar Pradesh, India, 1991. BOTTOM: Ray crossing the Ganga in Mayapur, West Bengal, India, 1988. OPPOSITE TOP LEFT: Bhakta Tony at the Holi festival in Vrindavan, Uttar Pradesh, India, 1991. OPPOSITE TOP RIGHT: Ray reading stories of Krishna to locals on a 24-hour train trip to New Delhi. OPPOSITE MIDDLE: Ray at Gariahat Market in Kolkata, West Bengal, India. OPPOSITE BOTTOM: Ray, Bhakta Tony, and Bhaktisvarupa Damodara Swami with members of a local metal band in Manipur, India.

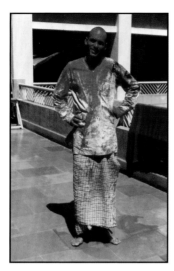
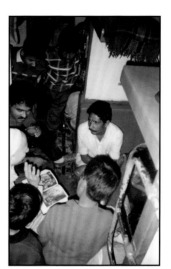
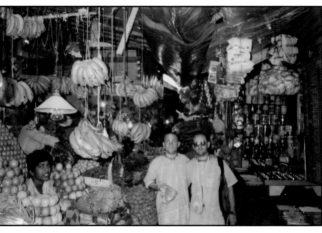
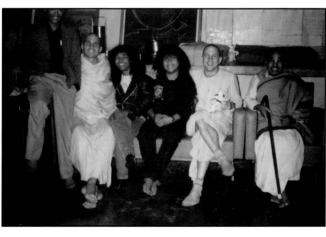

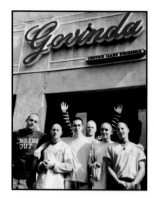
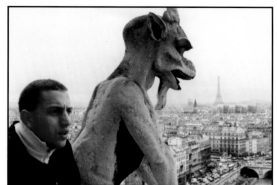
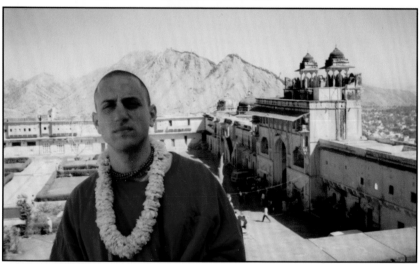
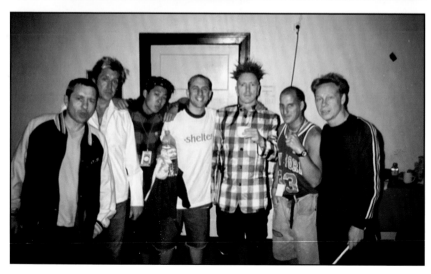

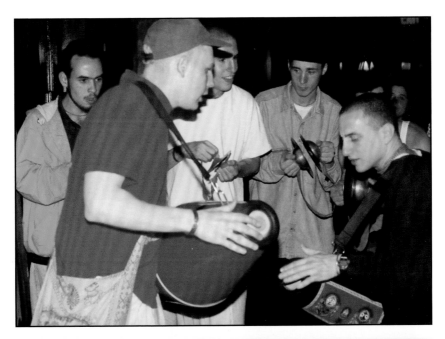

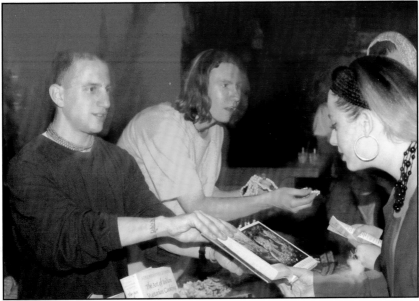

OPPOSITE TOP LEFT: Shelter at Govinda restaurant in Milan, Italy, 1989. OPPOSITE TOP RIGHT: Ray at Notre-Dame de Paris in Paris, France, 1989. Photo by Jordan Cooper. OPPOSITE MIDDLE: Ray in Rajasthan, India, 1991. OPPOSITE BOTTOM: Shelter backstage with the Sex Pistols in Berlin, Germany, 1996. Photo by Pedro Nicolas. ABOVE: Ray leading kirtan and selling the *Bhagavad Gita* before a show at the Limelight in NYC, 1992. Photos by Lenny Zimkus.

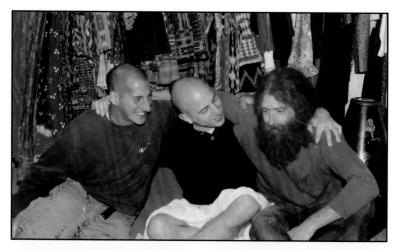

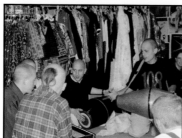

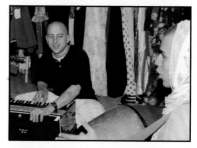

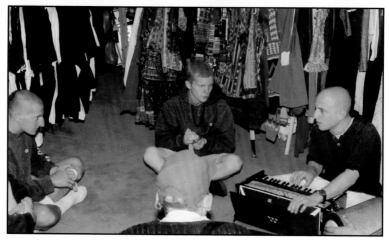

ABOVE: Ray and Porcell reuniting with Warren from Violent Children for an in-store appearance at Trash American Style in Danbury, CT, 1993. Photos by Lenny Zimkus. OPPOSITE TOP: Shelter mixing *Attaining the Supreme* at Don Fury's recording studio in NYC, 1993. Photo by Ray Lego. OPPOSITE BOTTOM: Creek swimming and outdoor kirtan while on tour in Grass Valley, CA, 1993. Photo by Lenny Zimkus.

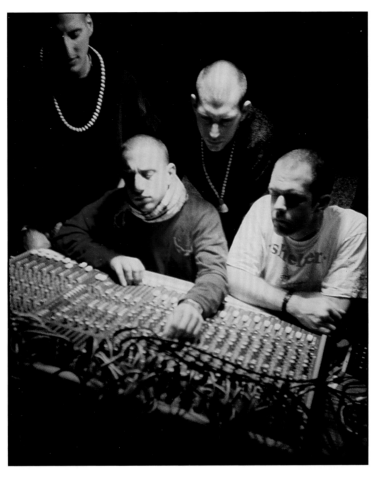

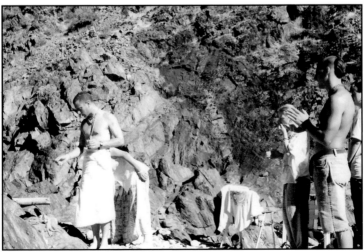

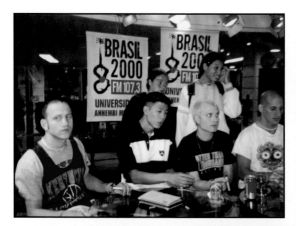
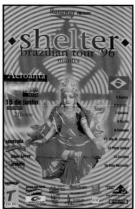
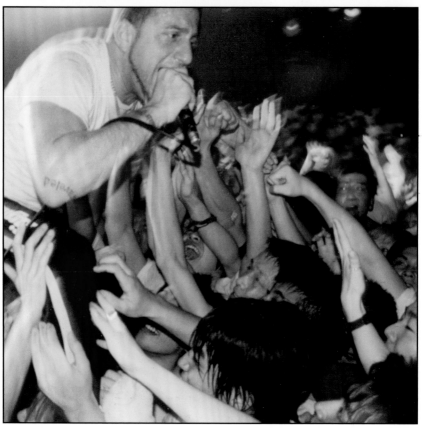

TOP LEFT: Shelter signing autographs in Brazil, 1996. TOP RIGHT: Brazilian tour poster, 1996. BOTTOM: Shelter performing in Tokyo. OPPOSITE TOP: Ray singing with Gwen Stefani when Shelter opened for No Doubt, 1996. OPPOSITE BOTTOM: Shelter performing at Irving Plaza in NYC, 1995. Photo by Chris Tolliver.

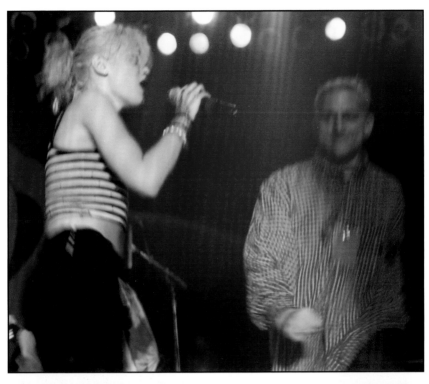

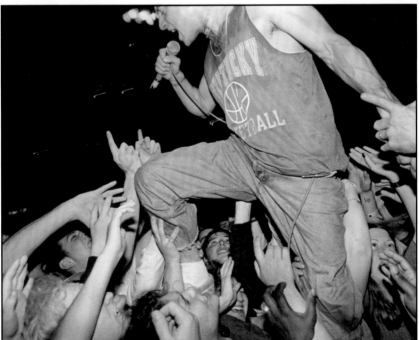

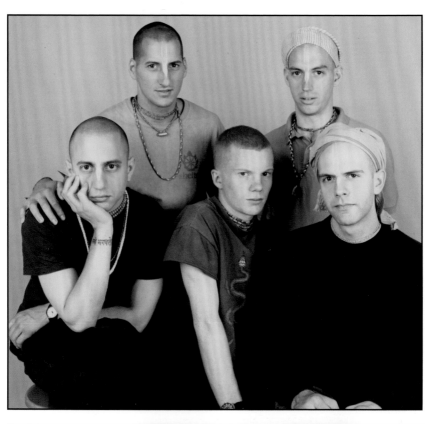

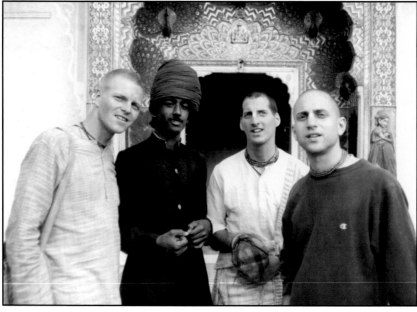

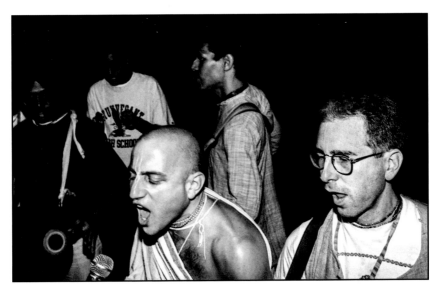

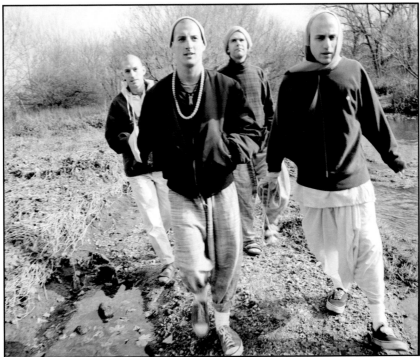

OPPOSITE TOP: Shelter, 1992. Photo by Jerry Klineberg. OPPOSITE BOTTOM: Ray, Porcell, and Steve Reddy (Equal Vision Records) in Nathdwara, Rajasthan, India, 1993. TOP: Preshow kirtan with Norman Brannon and Hari Kirtan, 1993. Photo by Ray Lego. BOTTOM: Shelter, 1993. Photo by Ray Lego.

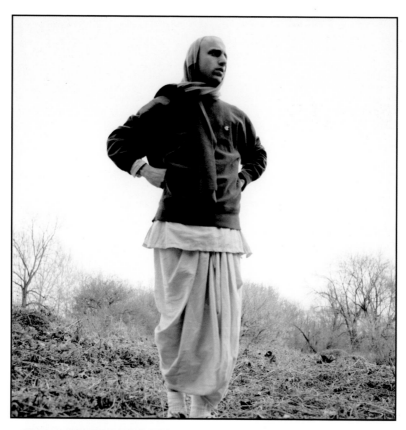

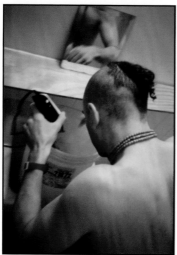

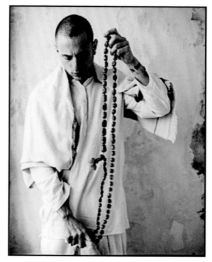

ABOVE: Ray at ISKCON Philadelphia. Photos by Ray Lego. OPPOSITE: Shelter at
ISKCON Philadelphia. Photos by Ray Lego.

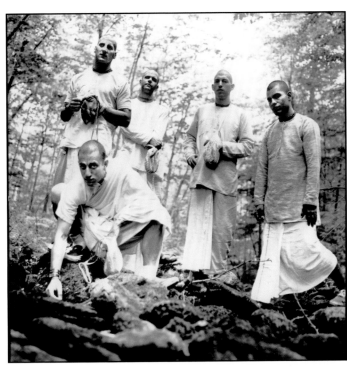

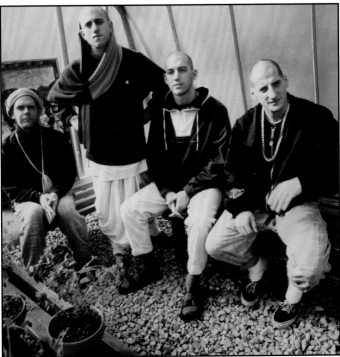

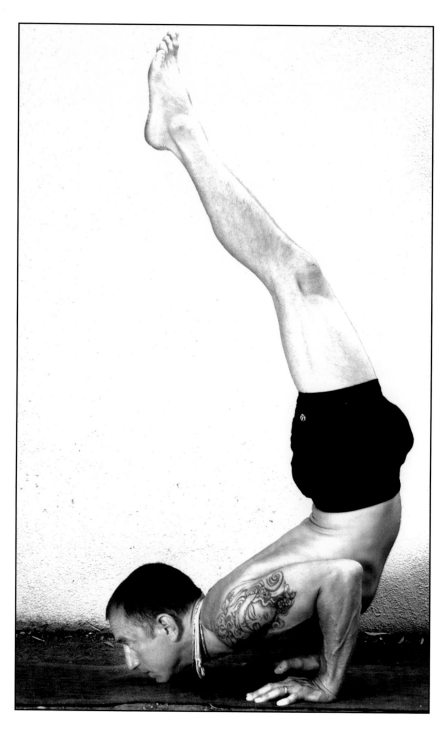

ABOVE: Ray in ganda bherundasana, 2000. Photo by Eye of Laksmi Photography.

"This is important stuff, Ray. It's changing the way people treat other living beings. This is great news."

"Thanks. But I quit. I mean . . . I just need God at this point in my life."

"That makes sense, too," she said, nodding. "I have to record now. I hope we can meet up again. I'll be at the temple tomorrow around the same time."

"That would be incredible. Thank you. And thanks for what you do."

She went into the recording studio, and I stood there in awe. I met her the next day for a similar excursion and thanked her for coming into my life as a messenger and giver of truth. I held on to her words.

*   *   *

My taxi pulled into Vrindavan in September 1988. I stepped out of the car and breathed deeply to slow my heartbeat. There was a strange aroma in the air. The smell of incense, diesel fumes, and burning cow dung gave me a new sensual experience. It was 8:30 a.m., and the sun was already warm. The red bougainvilleas lining the temple gate were brilliant firetruck red, and the air was dry.

The car ride from Delhi was unnerving. The driver had one hand on the wheel and the other on the horn the entire way. It was a sonic assault. A four-hour nonstop Morse code of a honk. He drove at breakneck speeds over unmarked potholes. He swerved for a camel cart, dodged three water buffaloes, threw me side to side in the back seat. The paved road occasionally switched to dirt, sending me up and down like a piece of cargo. Then, without warning, the driver would slam on the brakes for a shepherd leading forty goats across the street.

"Jai Sri Krishna," the driver said in a new state of peace and euphoria. It was obvious he was also deeply connected to Krishna and this holy town. A small statue of Radha and Krishna was glued to his dashboard. "Sri Vrindavan dhama. You have arrived." He gave me a sweet smile and head bobble. He seemed totally unaffected by the trauma I had gone through. Just business as usual.

I reached into my pocket and pulled out rupees I had exchanged for in the airport. He took them in his hands, which were already in namaste, and smiled and head-bobbled again. Next, I reached into my other pocket for the crumbled piece of thinner-than-paper airmail that confirmed my reservation for the Vrindavan guesthouse. I didn't see anyone standing behind the desk, but as I moved closer, I noticed a man covered with an Indian shawl sleeping on a bench.

"Hare Krishna," I said loudly to wake him. "I have a reservation. My name is Ray Cappo." He quickly got up and assisted me. I heard kirtan from the temple's morning program, and somebody walked in wearing the biggest flower garland I had ever seen, spilling rose petals on the floor behind him as he walked. The scent of those roses filled the room. Older Indian ladies in saris walked up the stairs toward the guest rooms, looking like Indian royalty and chattering away in Hindi while eating sweets out of five-inch leaf cups. Right outside the entrance, a woman screamed. When I turned, I realized a monkey had taken a tangerine from her hand and was making a stealthy getaway. I paused and looked around. Where was I?

* * *

I wasn't sure when my brahmacharya studentship would end, but I knew it was my calling for now. This is the traditional celibate student life of service to God. Truthfully, sexual abstinence was a relief for me. I had known for a while that there was no person that could give me what I needed. No human who could make me whole. No soulmate could fill the God-shaped hole in my heart. I was sick of the concept that there was another person out there who would make me complete. So I turned off my sexual urges. And there are techniques to do so. No touching. No looking. No hanging out with girls. No dallying or joking with them either.

"What's wrong with hanging out with girls?" I asked an older monk. "After all, we're all spirit souls."

His answer was short and simple and made sense. "Yes, you are a spirit soul. But there's no time you are more convinced that you are a man than when you're hanging out with a beautiful woman."

To be a celibate monk in my twenties wasn't an easy task, but I held firmly to my commitment. If my mind was attracted to someone, I'd tell myself mantras such as "Beautiful but not what I need" and "Externally beautiful but will not give my heart what it needs" and "Pleasure is fleeting. Find the eternal pleasure."

I struggled with it in my mind to be honest. We grew up hearing that men think of sex every seven seconds. Researchers now say this is much exaggerated but still conclude that a good romp goes on in a man's mind about every hour and twenty-six minutes. But I was learning to cultivate a condition by practicing what I was thinking. Some people chose not to think sexual thoughts. Some people choose to indulge in them. Some people run on autopilot according to their predisposition and the company they keep.

I had been one of those on autopilot. But by this point in my life, I had realized that lust could possess one's mind. It was magnets and metal. Even as I lived in the ashram, when my head hit the floor to sleep, these fantasies would appear. They were hard to get rid of, even when I knew these things were dreams that wouldn't give me what I wanted. As soon as I tried to harness my mind, I realized how much my mind owned me. But as I got stronger in controlling my thoughts, my mind got weaker.

I had a bad attitude. It was part of the reason why I started my spiritual journey. I had eliminated drugs, alcohol, cigarettes, and animal flesh from my life. I felt a strong calling for internal cleanliness and got obsessed with health. But my bad attitude got the best of me. Now on this journey through sacred India, my bad attitude was getting more and more obvious. I didn't like what I had become. I proclaimed a positive outlook on life—in my song lyrics, to my audience. I knew it was important to trust, to see the good, be kind, loving. I got it. And it was in me. But it was eclipsed by darker forces.

Internally, there was a heavy dose of cynicism that was running through my blood, mixed with a double shot of sarcasm. I held grudges. I was easily offended. I'd double down and attack if I was criticized. I was fearless and could take to violence if threatened. I was often envious of others' good fortune. All of this is embarrassing to reflect on now, but it's the truth. And it was time to do some real inner work. Mental modifications. Or else I'd never find peace or connection in this world.

I was starting to realize that these problematic thoughts—lust, greed, envy, and competition—were made worse by any success I had in the band. Music success seemed like a great thing, but it heightened these darker emotions. I'd feel *more* competitive, *more* self-righteous, *less* tolerant, *more* arrogant, *more* entitled, and thus . . . *more* sad. These were the biggest demons I needed to slay.

* * *

After a few weeks of living in the guesthouse in Vrindavan, I moved into a small, square, cement room. A few young Indian men and I slept on the cement floor on top of bamboo roll-up mats. I also had a puffy American sleeping bag. Living in the ashram conditioned me to wake up early. I'd roll up my sleeping bag, wash the area on the floor where I slept, then wrap my waist with a gamcha (a thin cotton towel). I would take a second gamcha, shove my neem chew stick in my mouth, and head to the bathroom with my toilet essentials. The bathroom was prisonlike. Dark. I scraped my tongue with a U-shaped piece of copper. We were taught that the body released toxins through the tongue as we slept and the first thing we should do was scrape our dirty tongues. Some monks stuck it way back in their throats, so the gag reflex became audibly loud in the communal space.

Then I'd go to the toilet. The toilet was a squatting toilet. No seat. No bowl. Just a hole. I had to relearn how to defecate, as strange as that sounds. I loved it. Two porcelain bricks for each foot were on either side of a lightbulb-shaped hole about one and a half feet long. I'd take my gamcha off, squat, and hover over that hole. Three-fourths of the world's population pass stool like this. The sitting toilet is a modern contraption that has proved to be problematic for a healthy elimination of the bowels. Why do you think we have so many books and magazines in the commode in the United States? We're living in a constipated culture. Many Ayurvedic doctors say that disease begins with poor elimination. Squatting stimulates the apana vayu, or the downward flowing wind of the body, which is perfect for defecation (and childbirth; the Western way—lying on the back—is considered unnatural and counterintuitive).

There was no toilet paper, another modern invention. In India, toilet paper was considered unclean. If you stepped barefoot on dog crap, you'd probably use soap and water to wash your feet, not wipe it with a piece of paper. Likewise, you were expected to shower every time you defecated. A small steel lota—shaped like a roundish cup with a lip—was placed in every toilet next to a spigot in the wall. You poured the water down your backside, using your left hand to wipe. Fortunately, the squatting process opened the bowels up, resulting in a less messy wiping job. After washing my hands, I'd put my gamcha back on and head for the shower.

The showers were pretty jailhouse, too. Spigots came out of the wall, and there was nothing but an on-off lever. The water was stored in a tank on the roof. It came out super cold in the winter and fiery hot in the summer. I braced myself for the cold, smiling and chanting, "I'm not the body, I'm not the body." Keeping on my gamcha and Brahmin underwear—two strips of cloth that held the genitals down and tied in the back—I submerged myself in that cold water and lathered my Chandrika-brand Ayurvedic soap all over my body. Then I removed the wet underwear. I felt strangely warm when I got out of the cold shower. I was taught that cold showers were good for my body's constitution, strengthening my immune system and my circulation. I washed my underwear after bathing and wrung them out. (I had two pairs of underwear. They dried within a few hours.) Then I turned off the spigot, got my dry gamcha, and wrapped it on top of the wet one while simultaneously removing the wet one. Civilized people always kept their private parts covered, even in private.

Then I wrung out the wet gamcha and dried myself off with it. The wet gamcha got rid of most of the water on my body, and the air dried the rest. There were no big, fluffy towels in the ashrams. They were considered unclean, as most people did not wash them after every use. Gamchas were rinsed with water and left to dry in the sun, deeming them suchi, or clean to use. One of the monks told me that water purified cotton, wind purified silk, and wool was always considered pure.

*   *   *

"Meet me in my room at exactly 4:45 a.m.," said the sober-minded monk, or my Swami-ji, as I called him. Swami-ji was an older American monk who had come to live in Vrindavan many years back. After university, he gave his life to the ashram in the 1970s, when the early stages of the Western Krishna movement seemed more regimented and extreme. I missed that era, thank God.

Although there were teachers and administrators who were obviously held in respect in the ashram, Swami-ji was simple, and I could appreciate that. His renunciation was joyful. He looked after me like a father figure, which was incredibly therapeutic considering my father had just passed. He lived like all the students. He slept on the floor, and at a certain point he invited me to sleep next to him in the office he had. I was struggling to adapt to Indian living, and he showed extreme kindness and tolerance toward me. Like me, he slept on a mat in a sleeping bag. He took cold showers, and he enjoyed serving the prasad during the mealtimes.

What I loved most about him was that he refused to find fault with anyone. He warned me, saying it was the major reason why people leave their spiritual practice. "Lord Krishna will not tolerate people who are rude to his devotees," he told me more than once. "Never find fault—it is spiritual suicide." I never heard him speak ill of anyone, even when I knew some people may have bothered him. He always saw the good and spoke kindly. His saffron robes were not fancy They were cheap cotton. Sometimes the gurus or swamis had beautiful silk robes, gold rings, and watches given by adoring disciples, which triggered my cynicism. *Who are they kidding with a gold watch? I would think. Who are they trying to impress? Why would they care about that? They're supposed to be renunciates.* They would justify those indulgences with phrases like "We're preachers, and we should look presentable" or "I'm honoring a gift, and it's good for the disciple to serve the guru" or "It's a good watch. There's nothing sinful about having a good watch. Be practical."

But I didn't buy it. Swami-ji had a Casio. A Casio so crappy that even I wouldn't wear it. And Swami-ji had no air of importance. He even wore the robes I'd burned while ironing them. His broken spectacles, which he needed to see, were taped together. He was a simple monk and an excellent teacher.

Most of all, he had a childlike fascination for Krishna and would sit me down and show me pictures of temples and read to me from books. "Look how beautiful Krishna is, Ray!" he would say, opening up a book his guru wrote and pointing to a painting of Krishna and the cowherd girls. "Imagine seeing someone so beautiful in the material world. When we see a beautiful man or woman, sometimes we are stopped in our tracks. But Krishna is the source of all beauty, and he is breathtaking! The deer are in awe of Krishna as they just stop in their tracks."

I arrived back in the room at 4:45 a.m., after morning services. I wore my usual robe, high-top canvas Air Jordans, thick Wigwam socks, and a Champion hoodie. It was cold. I noticed Swami-ji's door was open. I peered in, and he was lying like a stick, face down with his hands reaching forward. A full prostration, in prayer, in front of his little altar. I walked quietly into the room so as not to disturb him and waited a moment. But he stayed down on the ground, not knowing I was in the room. More time went by. Twenty seconds. A minute. Two minutes. Three minutes he lay on the ground. I would have thought he was asleep, but he was mumbling something. I felt like I'd barged into his sacred space. When he rose, he was shocked to see me, but happy.

"Today we go on parikrama, Ray!" he said.

"What's that?" I asked.

"In the material world, we put ourselves in the center of everything. In the spiritual world, we take ourselves out of the center and put God in the center, and we do that deliberately by walking around a sacred place, temple, or deity. In this case, we walk around the sacred town of Vrindavan. It's about a two-hour walk. In doing so, we circumambulate five thousand temples." I was excited. I loved morning walks.

"Take off your shoes and socks and meet me on the grass," Swami-ji said. "You'll want your feet to touch the sacred earth. This is the same earth that Krishna and Balarama walked upon."

I quickly took off my high-tops and socks. "Oh my Krishna!" I said. It was bone-chillingly cold on the cement floor. I walked outside, and it was even colder, and dark too. "Swami-ji, I'm not sure I can do this," I said.

"You're really going to want the earth on your feet. It will affect you in a deep way. You'll get used to it as you walk."

Before the sun was up, we started our journey, but when my feet hit the sand, I couldn't take it any longer.

"I can't do this. It's like walking on ice. My feet are too tender! My bones are freezing. How do you do this?" I was bundled with a sweater, sweatshirt, winter hat, and long johns under my robes. I looked bizarre. I respected the holy traditions, but I couldn't pull this off, and was impressed he could.

Everything was cold and damp, including my bones. Swami-ji had nothing on but a small shirt and thin shawl. "Aren't you cold, Swami-ji?"

"Your body gets used to it. Like old farmers back home, you get a tolerance for the elements. When you're tolerant, you get stronger and complain less. When you complain less, you're less sad. This is Vrindavan life, Ray. Nobody around here wears shoes. They don't want to miss out on this sacred sand."

He picked up some sacred sand, which literally sparkled, and let it run through his fingers like in an hourglass.

I got it. But I couldn't do it. "I'm sorry," I said. "If I put shoes on, can I still go?"

"Sure," he smiled lovingly.

I took my socks and sneakers out of my bag, bent over awkwardly, and slipped them on. I walked behind him. The cold cut through my sweatshirt. I tried chanting on my mala, but I couldn't concentrate. The dark, moonless night, called Amavasya, made things extra dark, so I could barely see my hand in front of my face. The moonless night is considered very auspicious, as is the full moon, and many pilgrims came from neighboring villages and Delhi to walk around the sacred path of Vrindavan.

When we got to the official path, Swami-ji motioned to me to bow down. We bowed like sticks. Full prostrations. It was awkward for me, with rickshaws pedaling by. Then we started our pace. Swami-ji had quite a quick one to keep up with, considering he was older and barefoot. There was temple after temple after temple, each with congregants singing their morning mantras and prayers to their respective deities. It was charming, and the sweet melodies faded in and out as we passed the tiny ashrams. I peered into some ashram gates. Each ashram had its local devotees who went there to give up their worldly life or even retire. They shuffled around, mumbling mantras, slapping big hanging bells, or sitting quietly chanting on mala. I heard pumping water, which old men used to fill buckets and pour over their heads to take showers on the roadside. Even the poor were clean with frigid morning showers.

"Any one of these ashrams will welcome you in. You can wander right in anywhere. Don't be shy," Swami-ji said.

"They're all devotees of Krishna?" I asked.

"Yes, slightly different lineages, but yeah, they all worship Krishna."

Tongas, or horse-drawn carts, clopped by with drivers warning "Radhey, radhey!" I moved to one side. I heard the big bells of the temples ringing repeatedly, signifying that the arati ceremony had started. Some smaller ashrams were doing their morning services with softer bells that the priest rang in one hand while the other waved incense in circles around the forms of the deities of Krishna and Radha.

Herds of cows walked by unannounced, catching me off guard. If not for the bonging bells around their necks, the dark of early morning would have covered them completely, and I might have been trampled. I quickly dodged again. In the air hung wafts of rose and nag champa, or plumeria, incense, the smell of chai cooking in big woks, and of course the smokey, woody scent of dried cow dung burning in morning fires. Dung is a poor man's fuel for cooking or warming hands on chilly mornings like this one. Men squatted around the fire, rubbing their hands, drinking chai, and smoking cheap hand-rolled cigarettes called beedis. An occasional sadhu sat smoking hashish. I smelled the diesel of an early morning generator, which choked my nostrils.

I saw the silhouettes of monkeys, the same ones that created havoc in the daytime, sleeping in trees, quietly resting up for their morning mischief. Other pilgrims walked with me on this dusty trail, all barefoot except for me. We came to a blackish tree that grew out of a whitish tree. "This is the Krishna-Balarama tree," Swami-ji said. I squinted my eyes and noticed some light shining across the way. "Krishna is blackish, and his brother Balarama is whitish." The two trees looked amazing and even sacred. Many pilgrims went to the trees, touched them reverently with their hand, and touched their forehead to the bark in honor. Our walk continued down a quiet sandy path. There were remnants of ancient temples on either side of the road as if we were walking through kingdoms of ancient India.

"Vrindavan is not merely a holy place of pilgrimage," Swami-ji said. "It is called a dhama, a place that can give entrance into the spiritual world. But you cannot barge in. You must go in with a mood of service and humility. Then Vrindavan reveals itself to you. Not everyone is allowed that experience. And I've seen that Radha does not let just anyone enter. People can be here but not enter. This is the magic of Vrindavan. You cannot just buy a ticket here. You enter through love and devotion."

He continued walking and chanting on his mala. I followed.

We walked down a forested path and came to where aged brick walls had sacred peepal trees growing out of their sides, as if the jungle was taking over an ancient kingdom. Although I knew Swami-ji wanted to chant on his mala instead of talk, I couldn't help but ask, "How old is this place?"

"Well, Krishna was here five thousand years ago as a young boy, but in the ancient literature, Dhruva lived in this area. That was millennia ago."

"Millennia? Who's Dhruva?" I asked.

"Dhruva was a five-year-old prince who was sitting on his father's lap one day. His dad was the king," Swami-ji explained as we walked. "The king had two queens, and Dhruva's mother wasn't the favored queen. Dhruva's hostile stepmother pulled him off the lap of his father and told him he wasn't qualified because he wasn't born from her and only her son would be favored by the king. The king, having too much affection for this queen, did not protest and sent Dhruva away. Although Dhruva was a mere child, he was bent on revenge and went to a forest near here where he learned from yogis how to worship God to achieve success in his revenge. 'Lord Vishnu will grant all your desires,' said the yogi sage Narada, who was instructing him. 'Just repeat this mantra and meditate on Lord Vishnu within the heart.'

"The young boy achieved a divine vision of the beautiful form of Lord Vishnu after a very long period of meditation. Lord Vishnu's face was so beautiful, he couldn't look away. When he opened his eyes, Lord Vishnu was there and spoke to him.

"'What would you like, my son? I will give you whatever you like.' When Dhruva saw the beautiful smile of Lord Vishnu, his desire for revenge melted. Dhruva thought about why he had started his meditation. He wanted a kingdom, power, and revenge because his ego was hurt by his stepmother. Now, in this ecstatic trance, seeing this beautiful vision, he could say nothing at all, but simply smiled. He tried to speak but was dumb. Finally, he mustered up the words.

"'Lord, now that I see your beautiful face, I want nothing of this world. I came to this forest to do yoga and meditation. I wanted to develop a siddhi for power so I could use it to rule a kingdom of my own to prove my worth. I was searching for a piece of shiny, broken glass but in that search I found a diamond.'

"The demigods give people what they desire," said Swami-ji, smiling. "But Vishnu or Krishna is so beautiful, once you see his smiling face there's nothing in this world that seems attractive any longer. Do you know what I mean?"

I thought about my life. I did understand the exhaustion of material pursuits. I did understand that I, too, was materially exhausted and that nothing of this world could satisfy my heart. "I can imagine," I said.

I had glimpses of Krishna's beauty, and I believed this man had a taste for Krishna bhakti. Why else would a person live this austere life by choice? He wasn't getting sex or money. He had no position of respect compared to the other ashram swamis. He lived in a cement room with me and took cold showers and slept on the floor with me. He woke up at 3 a.m. to walk around a town barefoot at 4:30 a.m. He must have gotten *something* out of this. He was happy.

We began to glimpse the sacred Yamuna River. She flows south from the Himalayas through New Delhi and later through Vrindavan toward Agra, eventually joining with the Ganges and Saraswati Rivers at the sacred city of Prayagraj. At this holy confluence, the epic Kumbha Mela happens every twelve years, when literally millions of people bathe during Magha (January-ish) every morning for one month. It is the biggest spiritual festival in the world, and it has been going on since time immemorial. Swami-ji explained that the Yamuna, like the Ganges, was considered a goddess. She fell down from the spiritual world via the sushumna nadi, the subtle energy channel of the universe, manifesting at Yamunotri in the Himalayas, crossing through holy cities to the north, and arriving here in Vrindavan. The epics say she is the daughter of the mountain Kalinda and the brother of Yamaraja, the lord of death.

As we walked, the river became less visible. *She is perhaps older than the stars*, I thought. I noticed that many sadhus and holy people were moving toward her banks for a frigid morning dip. I could see boats on the Yamuna. Simple wooden ones, with no motor, just a boatman with a stick and perhaps an oar.

We arrived at Imli Tala, a massive tamarind tree. Lord Chaitanya would come for hours and chant japa under this tree. Swami-ji and I walked to the tree and circumambulated it. Swami-ji touched the tree then touched his forehead to its sacred bark. I copied him, and we departed.

The river started getting closer as we approached Keshi Ghat, a beautiful old palace with red sandstone stairs going into the river. Staggered chatras, or stone sitting places with umbrellalike domes, flanked the steps as they continued along the riverbank for at least a hundred meters. Sadhus would sit and study, read, or meditate under these chatras, and the roofs provided shade. There were no sadhus now, just mother monkeys fastidiously picking off bugs from their babies' bodies, just as a human mother would inspect her child's hair for lice. It was still mostly dark, and this daunting palace structure, guarded by monkeys, was basically built into the riverbank—both breathtaking and eerie. Monkey families delicately walked by on the narrow path between the palace and the river. Massive cows slept on the stone-trail steps, which led into the water, making the obstacle course even more challenging. A dark tunnel doorway appeared before us, as if we were stepping into a cave. It intimidated me, but the swami fearlessly led me in. I felt far from home.

A monkey screeched loudly, and I jumped, but in a moment, it was laughable. Then I was scared again for a moment as we crossed the sandstone steps with at least fifty monkeys on either side. Swami-ji reverentially approached the Yamuna River and taught me how to bow to her, take some water in my hands, and offer the water back to the Yamuna herself. With water cupped in both of my hands, I followed him, making clockwise motions in a gesture of love to the sacred Yamuna. Then we took more water and sprinkled it on our heads. Swami-ji smiled and said, "It doesn't get better than this, right?"

I agreed. There was something magical about all of it.

"Why do we offer Yamuna water to the Yamuna?" I asked. I never wanted to follow rituals without understanding the why behind them. "Why would the Yamuna, filled with Yamuna water, want us to offer her more of the same?"

Swami-ji smiled. "Yamuna is considered a great devotee goddess. Temples all over India offer Yamuna and Ganges water to their deities. You're correct—she does not need our water. What the great souls want to see is our love. Krishna, too, doesn't need our flowers. He's the very source of flowers! But Krishna loves our love. Krishna sees our love."

We climbed up into one of the chatras, which was perched ten feet above the rapidly flowing river. From this vantage point we saw the beautiful Keshi Ghat palace behind us, its stairs going down to the water, and could see Lakshmivan, the forest across the river that was filled with cottages, farms, and wild peacocks. I was in awe of everything—the architecture, the river, the small wooden boats, the old men chanting mantras, offering fire ghee lamps to the Yamuna, ringing soft bells, and singing morning prayers in high-pitched voices that were sweetly out of tune.

"Krishna doesn't need our offering," Swami-ji said, picking up where he left off.

We sat down on the sandstone steps to take in the beauty and so I could rest my feet. Behind us a massive temple of sorts ornamented the side of the river. There were little doorways that opened to temples of Krishna along the red stone walls. We walked through one doorway and sat down. It was a small room with cheap incense burning, like a big closet with an altar and a beautiful man sitting and chanting on mala. He spoke perfect English, although he looked as though he had walked out of the pages of one of the Indian epics. He had his hair tied in one big bun on his head. A white loincloth and a white chadar, or shawl, covered the top half of his body. His skin was oily and soft, and his big, full lips were cracked. He was old but had a childlike gaze about him. "Sit down," he said, gesturing, I could see his face through the crackling candle, and we got comfortable.

And after a few sweet exchanges, he told us a beautiful story. I was noticing that this seemed to happen a lot in India. This one was about Vidurarani and Krishna.

"Once, Krishna was visiting his great devotee Vidura and his wife, Vidurarani, who were quite elderly," said the man. "Vidurarani had so much love in her heart for Krishna that she meditated on him day and night. One night Krishna appeared at their home after a very long journey. He asked if she had any food for him. It was her dream come true—the lord of her heart manifested at her front door! She stood in trance, admiring His beauty. In her rapture, she forgot the appropriate ways to greet a guest. She didn't invite him in, offer him a seat, wash his feet, or even offer him any food or water. She just gazed at him awestruck, with love in her eyes. Krishna reminded her gently how hungry he was, and she shook herself out of her samadhi.

"'Oh yes, Krishna, whatever you like. Would you like some fruit?' Without taking her eyes off of Krishna's lotuslike eyes, she reached to one side and grabbed some bananas in a bowl. Then she started peeling the bananas. Again, in her rapture, struck by love, she mistakenly discarded the bananas and fed Krishna the banana peels. Krishna was shocked, but out of love for his devotee, he didn't want to bother her. He chewed those banana peels with great relish. He was tasting the love of his devotee and was satisfied eating the peels."

The story was sweet. I appreciated this, enjoying the early morning story time in a cavelike castle closet. My mind drifted to architecture. "Who built these beautiful old palaces?"

"Saintly kings from hundreds of years back would have holiday palaces in holy places," said the man. "They would build and maintain temples and guesthouses for their extended families and the priests. This was a vacation home for the saintly kings. Not only kings, but everyone would come to holy places with their families."

The sun was rising now, and Swami-ji and I rose respectfully and continued walking. In the distance, through a loud, low-grade PA system, we heard a call and response of "Hari om namah Shivaya" going back and forth between a man and woman. It got progressively louder as we approached their humble ashram. Ducking under a banyan tree, we bowed to a beautiful Shiva deity and continued our journey.

Pilgrims with quicker paces passed us, also doing the parikrama. Old ladies in saris, young men, families, little children, ladies holding babies. Some men wore traditional dhotis, and others wore knockoffs of Western clothing. It was cool to see this was a thing. People were taking the parikrama seriously.

"Some people make vows to do this every day for their entire life," Swami-ji said. "Every day going around. They can finish in two hours."

We walked through a quiet part of Vrindavan to sandy paths, farms, and tiny ashrams. More magic wherever we turned as we walked between random holy people, singing ladies, and stray cows. I was cold, but I felt healthy moving my body, even though I was still having trouble keeping up with Swami-ji. It was also hard for me to focus on my japa because I was looking around constantly. I wanted to stop for chai, but Swami-ji wouldn't have it. Chai, with its caffeine, was forbidden by the orthodox. We rounded the last corner and started the last quarter of the trail.

"You're moving a little slow, Ray, and I have to get back and prepare to teach some classes today," said Swami-ji. "I'm going to leave you here, but it's a straight shot from here to the ashram. You'll be able to see the big spires of Krishna-Balarama Mandir when you get closer in about twenty minutes. Are you comfortable finishing alone?"

I nodded. Swami-ji took off. The sun was risen now and started to warm me. I decided to take off my shoes and socks and put them in my shoulder bag, where they'd started before I caved to the cold. The town was officially awake. Kids were moving about getting ready for school, people were herding cows, there was more bustle on the streets, and the chai stalls became more crowded. The warming sun reassured me, as if saying, "Keep going, young man." I felt God was guiding me. I felt something shifting in me. I didn't understand everything, but I had a good overall feeling that I was going in a general direction of growth. My band seemed a light-year away. My old life seemed like a distant memory, almost like a dream. I started singing the *Mahamantra* out loud. Real loud. As if I was walking in a music video. I lifted my hands in the air in surrender to God's will. I sang joyously, praying. Nobody seemed to notice or care either way, so I just kept singing, smiling, and sometimes laughing for no good reason.

* * *

After bowing at the end of the trail, exactly where I started my journey, I dusted myself off and headed for the ashram a few hundred yards away. The very first person I saw was Swami-ji, who was standing effulgent in the morning sun, speaking to a student.

"Swami-ji!" I said, feeling grateful, smiling ear to ear. "That was such a wonderful morning! Thank you so much for bringing me on that transcendental journey. I feel so enlivened and fortunate! Thank you."

"You liked it?" he asked.

I nodded enthusiastically.

"Fantastic. For the next month, you should do it every day!"

I laughed nervously. "Oh yes, that would be great to do it every day. That would be wonderful . . . uhhh . . . but I have classes immediately. I don't think it would be practical to do it every day."

"Just make a commitment!" he said. "You'll get so much out of it. Vrindavan is a great place to make serious vows of service. And prayerful walks around holy places are a way we serve the dhama."

"I just don't think it would be practical." I smiled nervously. "But I really want to thank you for today."

Swami-ji nodded and walked off. Walking every day would be a lot. I was pretty exhausted from that walk already, and it was still quite cold. I felt a little unprepared.

As the morning ended and lunchtime approached, the monks started walking around carrying their metal plates. I became sentimental about my morning experience. To be surrounded by saintly people in a sacred town, with the sacred Yamuna, and to hear all those stories was a truly magical experience. I relished it. I turned around and ran into Swami-ji again.

"Swami-ji! I was just thinking about you! What a great morning I had. And when you left me there to walk back alone, I felt empowered and took off my shoes and just sang the entire rest of the way! What a beautiful way to spend my morning. Thank you again!"

"I'm glad you liked it," he said with a smile and nodding. "You should do it every day."

"Yes, every day would be amazing!" I said, feeling sort of awkward. This was now the second time I would have to decline. "But I just don't think it would work out for my schedule and my duties."

He dropped the subject and walked into the dining area, where people sat on the floor in two rows, facing each other.

"Are you eating?" he asked.

"Yes," I said. "I was going to go to the restaurant for lunch. I've got a little money."

"Ray, you asked me to give you advice, so that's the only reason I'm going to say this to you." He paused. "Do you mind unsolicited advice?"

"Well, I usually hate it, but I did ask you to instruct me while I'm here in this holy place," I said. "I want to make the most out of my experience. I want to understand the right way to enter Vrindavan."

"Don't eat at the restaurant. There's too much idle talk. Eat with the brahmacharis," he said. "Eat silently. Vrindavan is a place where Krishna is the enjoyer and we're the servants. Pleasure will come automatically from your service attitude. As a matter of fact, I've got a better idea. Don't even eat with monks. Serve them. I do it every day. I enjoy it so much. It's such a direct and simple way to serve the devotees. You get to nourish and lovingly serve each person. Make a commitment while you're in a holy place, a vrata, or vow. You're not here to be God. You're here to serve God and the devotees of God."

I could tell Swami-ji was trying to get me out of tourism consciousness and more into the experience of a sevaka, or servant, of the dhama and the devotees. I appreciated it. I didn't want to be a sightseer. I had asked him to instruct me in this regard, so I took it seriously and didn't go to the restaurant after that. I understood what he meant. I looked at Swami-ji and said, "You're right. Tomorrow I'll take the vow to serve every day instead of being served."

"You'll get a lot out of it," he said, smiling.

By the end of the day, I was inspired. One good action led to other good choices. I was happy Swami-ji encouraged me to serve lunch. It would be a nice way to tangibly take care of people. I felt like my appetite was strong and healthy after that divine walk in the morning. I started to reminisce about the sounds and smells of the morning and inwardly smiled. Then, as if magically, Swami-ji appeared again.

"Swami-ji!" I said. "So crazy I was just thinking about our morning parikrama. It was so special." I was as enthusiastic as I was in the morning.

"Really? I'm so glad you liked it. You should do it every day." That was the third time he told me to do it. The first two times, I had dodged his request, making excuses. Now, slightly inspired, I took this as a divine harbinger of good fortune.

"Yes. I will do it every day."

* * *

I woke up at 3:30 a.m. on the floor next to Swami-ji's room. He was already awake, chanting quietly on his beads. I took my cold shower and got dressed, and when I returned I started reading from a book I had bought that describes all the holy places along the parikrama trail. It was almost like getting a treasure map with insider info. After the morning kirtan in the temple room, I quickly darted out of the temple gate, performed my prostrate obeisance at the trailhead, and headed off in the early morning cool fog. I tried to keep a quick pace and follow the basic guidelines (although I kept my shoes on). I bowed and touched the Krishna-Balarama tree, as I had seen others do. I also touched wandering cows, and then put my hand to my forehead, signifying respect for their sacredness. Occasionally, I touched the sand, also known as brajraj, or the sacred dust of Vrindavan, which is said to give one bhakti within the heart. I sprinkled it on my head.

Day after day I'd bring songs to learn and sing out loud, as well as chant on my mala. I'd wander deliberately into one of the many hundreds of ashrams along the trail. Each was inviting, friendly, and charming in its own way. I'd meet the holy people of that ashram, speak to them in my broken Hindi, chant with them, and sometimes sit and eat with them. The atmosphere on the trail changed as the moon waxed. The trail was less eerie when dominated by moonlight. On certain holy days the trail would be packed with pilgrims. Sometimes ladies in packs of ten to fifteen would walk by, singing songs and clapping. Solo sadhus would zip by carrying a protective monkey stick. Or teenage boys, perhaps from Delhi, would walk by laughing. I thought about American teenagers. They'd never wake up early to walk around a sacred town. As brash or as loud as some of the teenagers on the trail were, they were devoted, sweet, and impressive compared to the teenagers I grew up with.

And they were all barefoot. Occasionally, a sadhu would see me walking and disapprovingly point to my shoes, shaking his head. I pretended I didn't understand, but I understood. He was telling me to take them off. In a week, I took off my socks. And in ten days, I started barefoot. That first day was the most difficult. Parts of the paved road were bad in the cold, but the cold sand—that was torturous. After a few days my feet hardened. They became like leather, shoes in their own right. I felt like a Sherpa. Each day was a new adventure with a new cast of characters. One day I got robbed by a monkey. Another day a pack of dogs chased me. Some days I met a saint.

* * *

I had an incredible realization and experience when I took my vow to serve lunch, or prasad. Swami-ji took the lead and started instructing me. On my first day, he had me meet him fifteen minutes early. There were about three hundred people eating at once, sitting on the floor in rows facing each other. Each had their own metal mess-hall plate and stainless steel lota, or roundish drinking cup. Ladles and buckets with fresh preparations were brought to the front of the line. Each bucket was covered with a cut banana leaf. The buckets contained a subji—a curried vegetable preparation—rice, dal, and fresh chapatis with ghee, which had been cooked on open flames. It was a delicious meal. Swami-ji explained the science of serving, which I found fascinating.

"You see how there are two rows facing each other?" he said. I nodded. "Never serve one side first and then the other." My face made a question mark. "Always go back and forth down the row. If you serve one side, the other side becomes envious of the others' prasad. That glance of envy contaminates the food. Always serve back and forth and as quickly and cleanly as possible.

"We have a team of servers, and you have to be closely serving together. We never want the devotees to have to sit there with a pile of rice and be waiting for the subji or dal. We want to do this with love and efficiency, so they're happy and pleased and have good digestion. They shouldn't ever be looking around, thinking, 'Where is that brahmachari with the dal?' Those who are eating should never be thinking, 'Where is *this* preparation? Where is *that* preparation?' Preparations should be brought to them before they can even think about asking for anything. Their only reply, as they're eating in silence, should be to keep their hands on their knees, which means they want more, or to put their hand over their plate palm down, which means they've had enough. If their hand does not go over their plate, you continue spooning the prasad on their plate until their hand rises. They should never feel like you are holding out on them. Always make them feel like there's plenty of prasad and that we will not run out. Never make them agitated and needy. Our mood is service.

"The servers start with anything that will not get cold. Today, we have chutney and pakoras. That should be quickly put on everyone's plate. The dal stays hot the longest, so that should be next. Nobody should be getting cold prasad; it ruins the digestion. Next would be the subji. Because it's water-based, it will also stay warm, and the rice is served last because it cools off quickly. Chapatis are served as quickly as possible after the kitchen servers bring them out. Nothing is better than a hot chapati."

I could tell Swami-ji loved this service, and his excitement was getting passed on to me.

"When all the preparations have gone around three times at least, then you go to each person with folded hands, look them in the eye and say, 'Can I serve you in any way, Prabhu?' or 'Is there anything else I can get you, Prabhu?' This will make them feel really taken care of. If they say no, you step to the person next to him and say the same thing. At that point, people will be leaving and clearing their plates and washing up outside."

"Do we put food aside for us in case we run out of prasad?" I asked nervously. "How does that work?"

"Some servers do, but I don't," he said. "I don't recommend it. I recommend telling yourself if we run out of prasad, then we will skip that meal and see it as a wonderful chance to serve the devotees. Once we have the scarcity mentality that Krishna will not take care of us, we will be stingy with our service. Let's just trust."

My face froze up, as I was hungry already. *But yeah! Why not! Just trust!* I thought.

We served each preparation meticulously. I started following the dal guy around with the subji, and the rice guy was close behind. The servers didn't speak, but just made gestures or occasionally said something in Hindi, such as "chawal prasad" or "dal, dal, dal." For the most part, we were as quiet as were they. The serving team was efficient and quick, and Swami-ji directed it and served alongside us. I could tell he took great joy in the systematic way it was executed because everyone appeared very happy. This made him happy. The most satisfying thing was seeing everyone fed to their fullest. I knew they were satisfied because they put their hands over their plates, palms down slightly, waving them back and forth when I came around with my subji. They were stuffed. Blissful. And to my joy, there were plenty of leftovers. Then someone brought in a massive plate of mahaprasad from the altar, filled with samosas, chutney, bitter melon, sweet rice, and puris (round white-flour tortillas thrown in woks of ghee until they puffed into a perfect ball). It was like a Krishna reward for being good! I smiled and felt great for this simple yet satisfying service.

As I served each day, I grew to enjoy it even more. When people sat down to eat, they immediately got possessed by an attachment to enjoy, and they could be a little irritable. It became my joy to pacify them with a quick and efficient service. The most pleasurable part of it was to go to each person with folded hands and, in a sweet gesture, say, "How else can I serve you, Prabhu?" These relationships made me begin to fall in love with Vedic culture. Sure, it was philosophical. Yes, it was deep. It was thoughtful. It was grave. It was steeped in culture, but most of all, I found the underlying sweetness, devoid of any ego, attractive and heart-opening.

"Humble like a blade of grass," Swami-ji would say. "Not looking for respect, but ready to give it, to whomever you meet. Tolerant like a tree. These are the teachings of Chaitanya Mahaprabhu, the Kirtan Avatar. These practices make your chanting go deep. This serving of prasad to the devotees is a way to develop those qualities."

I thought about my previous life in New York. I didn't drink, smoke, take drugs, or eat animal products, but I didn't have this sweetness. I was riddled with ego. Like a disease. I was arrogant. Rather than being sweet, my dealings with friends were usually sarcastic, cutting, and rude. I wasn't sure how I got so offtrack.

"Not looking for respect, but ready to give it to everyone. This is the secret of the entire bhakti yoga system," said Swami-ji. "This is the secret of life. Then the mantra becomes part of you and transforms your life!" Swami-ji was smiling and inspired, and that made me inspired.

* * *

I continued walking around Vrindavan every morning, and I found it quite joyous. Each day was magical. I felt connected, healthy, and adventurous, roaming into new ashrams and meeting interesting holy people. But one day I woke up feeling down. There was no good reason for it. Everything was going well. I liked what I was doing, but my mind told me, "Today is going to suck."

From there, I searched for evidence of how it *would* actually suck. I thought about my cold shower. I didn't want to do it. I thought about putting on my dhoti. It always ended up falling off me. I didn't want to wear it. I thought about the morning kirtan. No, I didn't want to do that, either. I thought about my freezing barefoot walk. No! I didn't want to do any of it, but I had taken a vow! I *had* to do it.

Still, I stayed in bed, procrastinating. Doubts about my life rose to the surface. *Why did I even quit my band?* I thought. The day before, I had received a letter from Porcell, the first piece of mail I'd received in Vrindavan. I was surprised and not even sure how he tracked me down. The letter read:

Ray,

Hope India is good. What's going on? What's your plan? Me and Sammy just got taken out to dinner by Michael Alago. Do you know who he is? He's the A&R of MCA records! He's the guy that signed Metallica! He may be interested in signing Youth of Today to a major label. What do you think? Are you into it? Everything is blowing up in NYC. Even the Beastie Boys are a household name now! It's unbelievable! Anyway let me know where you're at and when you're coming home. We hope you're having a good time over there. Don't lose your mind or give away all your savings.

Your bro,
Porcell

The Beastie Boys' rise to fame was pretty incredible. They went from nothing to a major-label success story complete with tour buses, professional road crews, international billing, television and MTV features, and adoring fans piling onto their tour buses. We had all been a bunch of punk rock hardcore guys with no ambition to be rock stars. We hadn't changed, but the music industry did. People wanted more powerful music, and my band was surely powerful and loud. The fact that Michael Alago courted my bandmates for dinner made my stomach drop. For a young musician, temptation didn't get any stronger than this.

The devil on my shoulder started whispering in my ear. "If you were world famous, then that hole in your heart would be filled," the voice said. "You think living in an ashram is going to fill that void? Who are you kidding? Buy a house. Have some fun. Live wherever you want. Have whoever you want. Finally people are appreciating your greatness! Don't waste an opportunity. Don't be a loser!"

I looked down at my robes and the mala in my hand. It was a Faustian offer for sure, and it was worth deep examination, especially since I had a miserable stomachache and diarrhea from eating street food the night before. I'd been keeping some golden mantras in my journal that saved me in times like these, where temptation sounded like a reasonable option. I opened my journal and pulled out a simple but effective mantra:

> *Think it through, Ray. Think it through. Think it through. Think the entire damn thing through. Think it. Think it through from beginning to end. You know too much now. Think it through.*

So I did: *You get signed to a big label. Do you know how many bands that get signed get dropped? Their hopes shattered. Not every major-label band ends up being Metallica. Most don't. They get a little money and then get dropped and it often ends their career and their integrity and their legacy in the eyes of the loyal fans.* Think it through. *Our band had a message of clean living, integrity-driven choices, and positive ideals. That was the force behind what we were doing. Now money is going to be the driving force? Fame is going to be the driving force? How much fame would it take for me to be satisfied? Can fame or money ever satisfy my soul? I'm already famous to some degree. That validation doesn't make me feel any more whole, connected, or grounded.* Think it through! *Do I just have to climb the fame stairway a little more . . . just a few steps more and then I'll reach some validation euphoria? Who cares about the validation from others if I love myself? These are tricks by maya. Illusion. Am I going to let fame and money kick me off my spiritual path? That's ridiculous.* Think it through, Ray!

Preaching to myself was powerful.

Still feeling a little melancholic, I skipped my morning walk. I skipped the entire morning program and stayed in bed. I decided to do my walking vow later in the day around 11 a.m. A little more than halfway through the trail, I got to the less-developed portion. This part of the trail was especially for sadhus, farmers, and simple ashrams, and it was like walking back in time. Sugarcane grew on the left, harvested by farmers and stacked into rickshaws and trucks, tied and bundled. Two little boys followed close behind, helping themselves to some canes that they bit, sucking out the sweet sugar sap and spitting out the fibers. True childhood joy. Cows meandered by, as well as a man playing karatalas and singing loud mantras and prayers, aloof to public opinion. He was walking this trail with me as a pilgrim. A water buffalo pulled a handmade wooden cart, which looked strange with its Firestone tires mounted on the axle, but it probably made for a smoother ride than wooden wheels. The cart was packed with grains and moving at the slow, steady, relaxed pace of the water buffalo.

Even with all this beauty, I still had a dark cloud hovering over my head. I was not sure why. Maybe it was frustrated desires. Isolation from old friends. Not having many peers around. Maybe the schedule I was on was too extreme. I continued my journey down the path.

The simple ashrams were built out of cob—dung, earth, and straw. Some were built out of cement. These were tiny dwellings covered with thatched or galvanized-metal roofing. There were miniature shrines and altars for the devotees of the small ashram to sit around on the hardened clay earth to pray, sing, or meditate. The earth was hardened by rubbing more dung and water on the earth itself in a circular motion. Afterward, the forest floor was even and as hard as stone, so it could be swept clean and maintained. Every three or four weeks, they redid the process to make it hard again. Many of these ashrams were in a row, one after another.

With my feet dragging and my head hanging, I saw a man sitting outside of his little temple structure on a marble stoop. He was beautiful, with a childlike smile and soft skin. The crow's-feet around his eyes revealed his age, most likely in his sixties. He was thin and dressed in rags—a tattered yellow dhoti, an old kurta that still had various colors on it from last year's Holi festival. He had a tiny unshaved goatee and long jet-black hair pulled back in a shikha. He had tilaks on his nose and third eye, and had sandalwood paste, which had been offered to the deity, smeared on his forehead as deity prasad. The sandalwood also helped him stay cool in the heat. The man saw me in my melancholic state and sweetly called to me as I walked by.

"Prabhu, prasad?" he said in a high-pitched voice, sweetly gesturing to ask if I wanted some sacred food.

I shook my head and put up my hand, gesturing "no thank you." I smiled and continued walking. I really didn't want to deal with anybody at that moment, but he insisted.

He folded his hands in namaste and spoke again while bobbing his head side to side. "Prabhu! Prabhu! Please, prasad."

I didn't know what to say, so I said something I might say in New York: "No thank you, I'm busy," even though I wasn't.

"Prabhu, please let me serve you."

I stopped and went over. He stood up to greet me with his beautiful hair and his beautiful face. "Please sit," he said, giving me his seat. I could tell he didn't speak much English. I sat. He faced his palms down at hip level and shook them up and down, signaling for me to stay where I am. His aging body climbed into a little room that served as a kitchen and came back with a small bowl of deliciously spiced chickpeas (chana), tomatoes, cilantro, and chilis. He extended his hands to me with the offering. "Please," he said.

I smiled, accepting. He immediately put the prasad down and quickly reached for a lota of water so he could pour it over my hands to clean them. "Pani," he said and motioned me to wash, as if we were playing charades. After cleaning my hands, I ate that delicious, loving bowl of chana. He smiled as he watched me eat.

"More prasad?"

I nodded. He immediately filled my bowl. When I was finished, he picked up the water for me to wash my hands again. "Pani? Washing?" We understood each other, and I held out my hands so he could bathe them for me. I felt honored. Then he looked into my eyes with deep compassion. There was a burlap mat on the hardened clay floor and a homemade pillow. He repeatedly touched the burlap mat with both hands and spoke in his high-pitched, broken English. "Lay down. Lay down, Prabhu," offering me an after-meal nap. His kindness and hospitality shocked me. I didn't move. I just looked at him. A smile deep down rose from my heart. *This is love*, I thought.

I lay down on my left side, according to the Ayurvedic practices I had learned in New York. I slept for about twenty minutes. Then I opened and closed my eyes, quickly stretched, and yawned. I saw my new friend sitting there, watching me. But it wasn't weird. He was like a loving parent.

I got up to leave and thanked him. "I'm very grateful," I said in English, touching my heart to help communicate that. "What is your name?" I asked slowly. He nodded back and said, "Hari. Bhajan. Das."

I paused and looked at him sincerely. "Thank you. Mera nam, Ray. *Raaay*," I said louder, hoping he would understand. "Shukriya, Hari Bhajan Das. Shukriya. Thank you."

I returned to the trail a changed man. My dark cloud was gone. It was amazing how this tiny offering of love spread to my entire being. *I want to be like that*, I thought. *I want to be like him. I want to learn how to love again.*

My face was beaming now, and I started singing mantras out loud, oblivious of the locals looking at me. I raised my hands in happiness and walked down the trail, smiling and singing like a man possessed by spirit.

* * *

The following day, I knew I wanted to go back at the same time to meet Hari Bhajan Das to repay him for his offering of love. I went to the mahaprasad stand at the Krishna-Balarama Temple where I was staying. The maha stand was a booth at the front of the ashram that sold little leaf or clay cups of delicious sacred prasad that had been offered on the altar. They were usually quite gourmet by American standards, but they were inexpensive and considered extremely sacred. I bought some chum-chums (tube-shaped milk sweets), kala jumuns (tennis-ball-sized spongy sweets with rock candy at their center and soaked in syrup), a samosa with tomato chutney, and a clay cup of saffron-and-cardamom sweet rice. I wrapped it all up in a little cardboard box and gently carried it on the trail, being careful to hide it from monkeys.

It was about noon when I got to his ashram, but Hari Bhajan was nowhere in sight. There was an older woman, plainly dressed, lovingly sweeping the earth with a handmade broom.

"Hari Bhajan kitar hai?" I said, asking if he was there.

"Hari Bhajan market. One hour," she replied in Hinglish.

"Oh brother," I said, sighing. I was an American. I didn't wait an hour for anything even when I had nowhere important to be.

"Please give these to Hari Bhajan," I said slowly. "From Ray"—I pointed to myself— "from New York!"

"No. No!" She was upset to see me leave after offering a gift and spoke in a pleading tone. "Hari Bhajan coming. He will come! Please. Sit. Please. Sit."

What could I do? The saintly older woman offered me a burlap-sack sitting place, so I parked it under the massive peepal tree, which shaded me from the sun with its gorgeous canopy. A peacock floated by. The old lady continued sweeping the hardened earth floor. I picked up my mala and started chanting. I was feeling like a real yogi sitting erect and looking out on the parikrama trail as pilgrims walked by barefoot and inspired.

Two men appeared out of the cottage where the ashram and kitchen were. It was nothing more than a hut, and these two looked like they'd been living there for a hundred years. They were dressed in rags, both with matted gray hair. They had about ten teeth between them. Their skin was weathered by the sun and old age, and the soles of their feet were thick from a lifetime of walking barefoot. I knew the soles of their feet because they both sat about eight inches in front of me. I tried not to be offended, but as an American, I tended to like my personal space. I was starting to realize that people here didn't have the same boundaries, especially in the villages. The two men stared at me.

"English bolte hai?" I asked.

"Ji nehi." Nope, they didn't speak a word. Their colorful-yet-worn plaid loongis, cotton cloths that wrap from the hips to ankles, were cranked up to their knees. Their smiles were big, and their eyes were beautiful.

Am I really going to have to sit here for one hour waiting for Hari Bhajan while these sadhus just stare at me? I thought. I tried to chant, but couldn't.

It was just too weird with people looking in my face, smiling, and nodding. You couldn't do this in New York City. People would get offended.

When I first arrived in India, I didn't understand the lack of personal space or the "space invaders," as I called them. One day I had gotten really offended. I was drinking a cup of hot lime water while talking to another visiting American. A young Indian devotee came up to me in the middle of the conversation, tilted his head steeply to one side, and just looked at me, like he was examining me—eyes fixed on me, getting close to my face. Like a good New Yorker, I just ignored him and continued my conversation. The gawker continued to gawk. I continued my conversation. But after a few minutes, this guy was completely staring, listening to our private conversation, and getting in my face. I snapped, threw my clay cup on the ground, and said, "What's up, dude? What's your problem? You got an issue with me? What's up?!"

My voice was loud and my posture threatening. I stood there, cocky and confrontational. He saw my fury and fearfully recoiled, apologetically drawing his head into his shoulders. He folded his hands in namaste and bobbled his head sweetly, with the countenance of a lamb. "I'm sorry, Prabhu," he said in a gentle, pleading voice. "I was just staring at you." As if that was just what he did.

I felt like a dirtbag, like the most offensive and nasty monk in the world. My New York conditioning had overwhelmed me. I immediately bowed down on the street and asked him for forgiveness. *I'm such a jerk*, I thought. *How did I end up such a jackass?*

So, this time, sitting at Hari Bhajan's ashram, I controlled myself. I decided to try another approach. "Karatalas, mridanga?" I asked, noting the two most famous musical instruments for kirtan.

That worked! They both smiled and one ran into the ashram and came out with karatalas and a mridanga. I took the karatalas and started singing the *Mahamantra*, and they eagerly joined in. The one who took the drum was adroit with his musical skills, and in short order, pilgrims started coming off the parikrama trail to sit with us and join in. Three ladies with brightly colored saris modestly pulled over their faces so I could only see their eyes and big gold nose rings harmonized during the call-and-response chanting. A family of five sat down. They looked like they came from Delhi, as the father was dressed in Western slacks and shirt. They politely sang along, clapping offbeat and doing the mantra backward at the wrong time, yet with enthusiasm and love. An old man carrying a stick doing parikrama sat down. He had no teeth, a shaved head except for his shikha, and a big, thick tilak of the South Indian tradition, with its red stripe in the center covering his forehead and nose. He had a smile on his face that could light up a room and began singing loudly, enthusiastically putting his hands in the air as if to signal "touchdown!" at a football game. Within fifteen minutes of starting the kirtan, we had at least thirty people join us, and it was probably the first big kirtan I had ever led.

Then it happened. An angelic dancing man in a high-pitched voice, two octaves higher than a normal man's voice, melodically screamed, "*Harrrrrrrrri booooooool!*"

It was none other than Hari Bhajan Das! He was dressed in his pale-yellow dhoti, with a matching yellow chadar wrapped aristocratically tight around the neck. He reached into his kurta pocket, grabbed some karatalas, and usurped my kirtan, leading it while dancing a jig that had me inspired. I couldn't help but smile. Hari Bhajan was a true showman. He kept this kirtan going on for about another thirty minutes and finally ended with auspicious prayers of gratitude.

"Sri Vrindavan dham ki," he called out.

"Jai!" everyone replied.

"Sri Yamuna Maiya ki," he called.

"Jai!"

And he continued, naming his guru, many famous deities and holy spots around Vrindavan, etc. The idea with the gratitude prayers, or prema dhvani, is that the leader remembers these holy people and places and the crowd calls out jai, which is the equivalent of hooray in English. Some British scholars translate jai as "victory," but I think hooray is more accurate, at least in the context of the prema dhvani.

Then Hari Bhajan Das went to the four corners of his ashram and said, again in his high-pitched, loud, singsong voice, "*Prasssssaaaaad!*" This signified that anyone who could hear him was welcome to come eat.

Suddenly, people started coming out of the kitchen with buckets of freshly made subji, rice, chutney, rotis, and cold drinks. It was an incredible feast. He had all the pilgrims line up, and he sat us down in rows. His students expertly served, and we ate until we were fully satisfied. Exactly as he did the previous day, he came to me after the meal and in a sweet, humble voice said, "Please. Lay down. Please. Let me serve."

And I did. I just lay down on the burlap sack, like I owned the place. Then I finally realized something. "Cul?" I said, meaning "Tomorrow?" He nodded. "Han-ji!" he replied, smiling. Every day at this time he served prasad to all the pilgrims. What appeared like a festival for me was business as usual for Hari Bhajan Das!

From that day on, I regularly ate with Hari Bhajan. His sweetness was contagious. I wanted to be like him. After lunch one day, I looked him in the eyes and thought, *Hari Bhajan, you are so wonderful. I want to be like you. I wish I could just have a conversation with you to find out your backstory.* Instead, our dialogue was more like a game of charades.

One day he looked at me with unpretentious eyes and spoke softly. "I am very small. I am very small. You are so great." He folded his hands.

I wanted to have a breakthrough with him. I wanted to get to know him. I wanted his story. I so wished I could speak Hindi. I cursed my ignorance. I felt like Hari Bhajan was a mysterious man with valuable information and life lessons to share. He may have had secrets of the universe in that joyous brain of his. Where was he from? Was he born here in this hut and inherited guruship from his father? What was his story? I made a desperate attempt to communicate with him.

"Do. You. Speak. English?" I asked, speaking slowly.

He looked at me confused. "Yes. Yes. Very much!" he said. "Since my childhood." I was overjoyed! Foolishly, I had assumed that he was uneducated or a villager who spoke a local language. I had been using hand signals and my broken Hindi on a fluent English speaker. "Hari Bhajan, where are you from?" I asked. "How did you get to Vrindavan?"

"I was a successful businessman in Kolkata," he said. "I had many people working for me. Money was no problem. I was not married and still very close to my parents. In my heart I always kept Krishna Bhagavan very close to me through the course of my workday. I'd read in the morning before work. I'd read before I went to bed. I was like a mother cow. Even while eating grass, the cow is thinking of her calf. This is how I would think of Thakur-ji," he said, using another name for Krishna. One day, my parents invited me on pilgrimage to Vrindavan. This was 1954. I was so excited to take this journey that I couldn't contain myself. When it was time to leave, I could not. In Vrindavan, everyone worships Krishna—the adults, the children, the birds, the trees. Even the earth and the ants. They are all doing seva with love.

"I looked at my parents soberly and told them, 'I cannot leave here.' My father smiled and said, 'Yes! Vrindavan is a wonderful place! How are we to leave? But we must catch a train in Mathura, so let us get a rickshaw and gather our things.' I spoke again with a dry, desperate voice. 'No. I cannot. I cannot leave this place. I will never leave this place.'

"My father was half-smiling, but looked puzzled and spoke seriously. 'You cannot be serious, my son. Let us go now before it is too late. I know you are attached to this wonderful place. I am also.'

"'No, Father, I will not leave,' I insisted. 'All of you go. I must stay. Krishna wants me to stay.'

"'But you have a career and a business! What are you talking about? Don't be capricious.' My father spoke now with a firm voice. 'You may have my business, Father. Sell it. Or give it away. I'm no longer interested in it. You may stay or go, Father, but I am never leaving this place.'" He paused and looked at me. "And I have been here ever since."

I was inspired. Sad for his father and family. But also awestruck. I saw myself in Hari Bhajan at that moment. *Of course!* I thought. There was no other intelligent answer.

"What do you do here?" I asked.

"I serve the pilgrims. Like you. I feed them. That is my service. My life is joyful. I miss nothing from my previous life," he said. "I miss nothing."

"How do you get money? How do you pay for existence?" I asked.

"Krishna provides. People see my seva and give me some money. I spend very little. Krishna provides for me. I am very small."

* * *

Be Here Now, by Ram Dass, is a classic book for Western seekers of Eastern thought. The title sounds great. We're living in our minds. We live in the future. We reminisce over the past and we cheat ourselves out of the present. The monk lifestyle I was living had me being here now. But it wasn't easy, and it wasn't fun. It was contemplative. I started to realize that most of my ideas of enjoyment were just that—ideas. I planned for happiness. I romanticized a particular life. I dreamed of a romance, a soulmate, to make me complete. They were all a plan to enjoy.

But that type of material enjoyment was merely a mental concoction. It was not based in the here and now. It existed in hope alone. I got that. But being here now was hard. The act of celibacy with my body and thoughts took me right out of the planning mind into the present mind. When my mind got lured by some possible future sexual enjoyment, my spiritual intelligence had to catch it and draw it back to my controlled self. Lust existed in the mind. Lust existed in hope for the future. It was not enjoyment in the now mind. It was a hope to enjoy.

In other words, my spiritual intelligence had to debate my senses and mind. *Don't live in the future. Be here now. That pleasure is not tangible. It is a hope in the mind. Therefore it is not real.*

Controlling the senses was difficult.

I had been in India for four months, living as a celibate monk and meditating for two hours a day. I was determined to keep these vows as I moved onto my next phase in life. I felt a loud calling for closure with my fans. I decided to head back home for Christmas to visit my family and focus on what I thought would be my farewell recording for my fans to explain who I was becoming and where I was going. I didn't know what my next step would be and was waiting for a sign. Would I go to an ashram in the United States? Go back to India? I made up my mind to leave India on December 23, 1988, but not leave my spiritual calling. I felt firm in my conviction.

* * *

I was going to head to Kolkata for some time and stay in the ashram there, and then to holy Mayapur in West Bengal. I had no set plan. I was just trying to let my inspiration lead me. My Vrindavan experience wasn't easy, but because it gave me so much, I wanted to leave appropriately in good consciousness.

I thought that my last day should be spent rendering service to a great soul. I knew that was an important facet of bhakti yoga. I knew an American monk named Kurma, who was dedicated to serving the cows and the land and chanting the holy name. I searched him out, introduced myself, and told him I was leaving Vrindavan the following day and that I'd like to be his servant for whatever he needed. He was amid cleaning up some land for the cows, which involved raking, picking up brush, and putting it in carts. I could do that. While I worked, I was able to ask him a few questions. I found that asking questions to people on this spiritual path helped me find my bearings. They gave advice about avoiding pitfalls and how to advance.

Sometimes, people thought monks were materially losers—monk life was an option for dropouts, guys who couldn't get a girlfriend, and failures. It was true that in some poor countries a destitute family gave their children to monasteries, an economic step up. They'd get meals, clothing, and even flush toilets. I saw this in some of the monasteries I visited. But this was not the case for the European and American monks, who often took an economic hit when they moved into an ashram. Many were from affluent families and university educated, and it was a massive sacrifice to move to an ashram in India where there's no hot water, you sleep on the floor, you have no possessions, you have no privacy, and you had to let go of the softness of American life. You did not upgrade your comfort level. Living in an Indian ashram was like camping out. I never felt refreshed.

Kurma was definitely not a loser. He looked regal. He was handsome, with a kind dignity in his face. He was cool to talk to and still humble and grounded as he raked the earth next to me.

"Kurma-ji, Prabhu?" I said, addressing him with reverence. "How did you get here? You appear to be materially capable, educated, attractive, down-to-earth. Why would you choose to relinquish all material joys that go with that good karma? What are you getting out of this? You're living with nothing out here, raking a field for cows in the middle of nowhere. Why? You look like you could do anything you set your heart to."

He stopped raking and looked at me, leaning on the rake almost like a cane or a staff. "I did have a great life, Ray," he said. "I had a wonderful girlfriend. But it was at the time of the Vietnam War, and I wanted to fight for my country. I thought it would be a good thing. The war was difficult. There was a lot of pain. A lot of unnecessary violence. No obvious enemy. And we weren't welcomed back as heroes. Not in the least. Many looked at us skeptically. The country was divided. I also had mixed emotions. I didn't fully understand that death could happen at any moment, but I did after the war. I wanted to get serious about my relationship with my girlfriend. We got married and moved to a beautiful place in Oregon, in a gorgeous part of the forest."

"Beautiful," I said, nodding.

"It *was* beautiful, Ray. I bought a small piece of land and decided to build my own house from foundation to finish." I was impressed. "There was a flowing mountain creek nearby, and I could channel that spring water right into my house, so my water was cold and fresh, coming directly from the mountains," he said, smiling.

"Oh, I love spring water!"

"My wife loved it, too. She gardened, so we grew our own vegetables, and we were both already vegetarians at that time."

"This sounds incredible! But it must have been cold, right?" I was trying to find some material flaw in the situation.

"Well, I worked for the forestry department, so they gave me the winters off. So, in cold weather, we'd fly to the Caribbean. We had a friend who had a house there that put us up, and it was a breathtaking way to opt out of the northwestern cold. The turquoise waters were our shelter during those bitter months, and when spring rolled around, we just flew back."

"That's amazing!" I said. But now I was dumbfounded. "Why would you give that up? That seems like the perfect life!"

"Because I knew in my heart it was all temporary," he said. "I had come across a *Bhagavad Gita* years before and kept it with me. The more I read it, the more I started to understand that no matter how well you can manipulate the material world to work in your favor, it's still just temporary. We are spiritual beings in a temporary world. I'd already seen so much death due to the war. I believe life has a goal. People were finding political goals, social goals, sexual goals, family goals, financial goals, but the *Gita* speaks of a spiritual goal while we're in this human body. None of the material goals will fulfill us because we're ultimately spiritual beings. The real goal is to reconnect with our Source. What's the big deal if I have a place in nature with spring water and vegetables growing? Even the deer and squirrels have that. Are we here for just healthy organic survival? What should I be doing? Just take up hobbies until I die? Do puzzles? It's all just buying time until we die. Don't you think, Ray?"

I couldn't say anything. He shattered my ideas, my hopes that maybe I was just doing material life wrong. Maybe things would be different if I just made a few adjustments. I still had hope in the material world. I hoped that there could be some lasting pleasure if I could arrange life deliberately to avoid pain and create a bulletproof existence where everything external worked out wrinkle-free. But Kurma already had that, and he said it didn't work.

"We live in this world trying to fall in love with things and people we cannot possess," he said, still leaning on his rake. "They will all be ripped away from us. We set ourselves up for great pain."

"So, what do we do? Not love?" I argued. "Not live? Give up on life? You could have lived in that cottage in the woods. Why did you have to leave that? It seemed good. It seemed right."

"It was good, Ray. My wife was good. My cottage was good, and the garden was good. It was all good. Maybe it was just me. It just wasn't enough. I had a louder calling. After the war, I felt like I knew too much. Nothing would be the same. I knew how fragile and delicate life was. That was the gift of war. It sobered me up to the fleeting nature of life. Once you start understanding your spiritual calling, once you listen to it, there's no going back to material life. Even sweet, sattvic material life. Comfortable material life. For me, that would have been burying my head in the sand. Pure escapism. I needed to be focused on my spiritual journey without distraction."

I was despondent and knew he was right. I was hoping there'd be an alternative, a shortcut, instead of surrendering to God. But the aching tooth cannot be ignored—it must be pulled. I was trying to placate and numb the aching tooth of material existence. I felt like Kurma-ji. I knew too much. I could not go back to music as I knew it. I was a caterpillar in hope of becoming a butterfly. That birthing process would not be easy or pain-free—it would dismantle my attachments, my persona, and the bravado that I had worked so hard to impress people with. But all of that was merely a costume to help me get by and get what I wanted. I wrote the following in my diary that night:

> *I've worn many costumes in my life already. I liked sports outfits so I could present myself as a sports fan to the world. I wore outdoorsman outfits to craft a personality of one who's connected with nature. I wore punk rock outfits to make a statement about how outlandish I was. Similarly, I had friends that wore preppy outfits and metalhead outfits to create some type of public identity. I've watched both myself and my friends change costumes again and again as we grew. Spiritual life isn't about wearing another costume (in this case a robe) to find our identity, it's about peeling off the layers of costumes to find our authentic self.*

I wanted to clarify something with Kurma-ji. "You're not saying everyone has to be a monk, are you?"

"No! No way, Ray. Most won't," he said. "Most will have families and take a more balanced approach to their spiritual life. Many will have that cottage and some kids. You have to do whatever you need to move forward on your path. This is just what I had to do, Prabhu," he said firmly. "And I wish you the best on your path." His smile was genuine, and he gave me a little namaskara with the rake between his hands, as well as a gentle head bobble. In a loving way, he pushed me toward a deeper trust and surrender, and made me realize the way out was in. Today was big.

* * *

Vrindavan was a dose of medicine too big for me to swallow. As much as I had this vision of nirvana in the holy land, I wasn't pure enough to be there. I knew this. There was something about this place that brought me very high and very low. Like a purging of lifetimes of karma in a few months. That holy place was like a makeup mirror enlarging my ego's blemishes. Instead of dealing with the blemishes, I paraded around like an arrogant prince. Yes, Vrindavan was crushing to that false ego, and on a few occasions it had me almost jump the fence back to my world of maya.

Vrindavan shook me to the core and made me face off with some serious demons I had no idea were living inside me. I didn't end up jumping the fence, but I was moving on from that sacred vortex to stay in an ashram in Kolkata. Still, the joy I experienced in Vrindavan was of the highest caliber. I relished new heights of realizations, the flowers, the beauty of seeing other soul seekers on their path, and the sweet people that loved me, took care of me, and inspired me over those four months. I would not soon forget the dusty town that became a magical home. Habits that I formed there—rising early, chanting, and meditating, singing, and dancing—would direct the rest of my life. Freeing my mind of media, consumption, and sex was a genuine relief and no challenge whatsoever. No, I would not ever forget Vrindavan, as a flying bird never forgets the nest that provides the deepest sense of comfort and home. Kolkata would be a more palatable dose of the medicine.

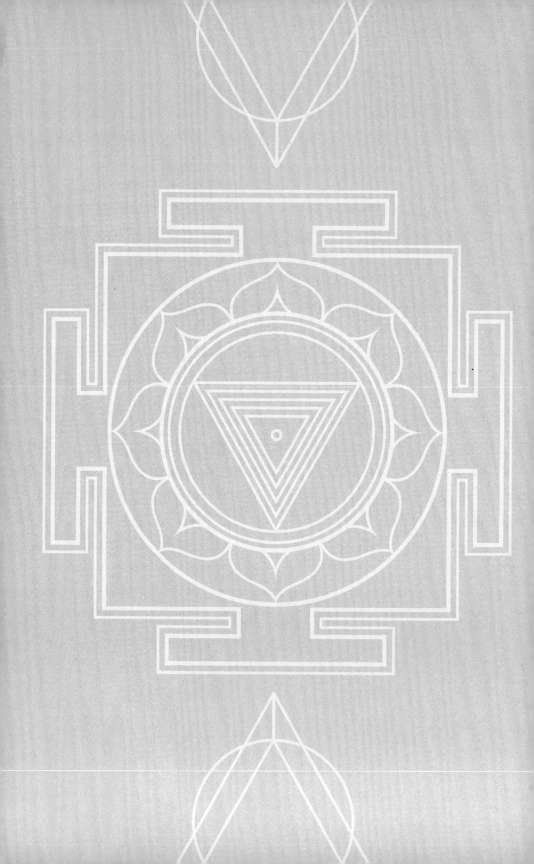

CHAPTER 7

KOLKATA

The heat never let up on that twenty-five-hour-turned-thirty-six-hour train ride to Kolkata. And even though I had been touched by the spontaneous chanting that Mohan had led in the train, I was still a work in progress and struggled with both my body and my mind for the rest of the trip, though I learned valuable lessons along the way.

When I couldn't stand the heat any longer, I bought a bottle of Bisleri, the only bottled water available. But it was as warm as the air and gave no relief.

Local Indians could drink anything. I saw them drink out of sacred ponds and rivers without incident. Not me, though. I would have gotten what some people called Delhi belly. I was delicate. One morning, I was singing in the shower at the Vrindavan ashram and tipped my head back to drink the water before I realized that I shouldn't be doing that. I ended up with dysentery for four days. No control of bodily functions. I had to sleep and live in the dark toilet with nothing but my gamcha wrapped around my waist. I brought in my journal and wrote because I had nothing else to do. Have you ever blown your nose so many times it becomes painful to the touch? My anus felt the same way for a week.

But the experience taught me about the material body. On the spiritual path, nothing is in vain. In one journal entry I wrote the following:

> *One forgets how miserable the body can become in a matter of moments. Some people live with chronic sickness and pain. I've been in pain now, and fasting, for almost four days and I'm complaining. How pathetic! With nothing to do, I begin to write. Durga, or Kali, is the Divine Mother and resides doing her seva in this material realm. She's what we would call Mother Nature, with all of her beauty and all of her fury. It's her service to Lord Vishnu to keep us in this material world of rehabilitation. In her expansion as Maya, she is the Goddess of Illusion, keeping all embodied souls lost chasing the temporary treasures of this world. It's that spell that keeps the foolish conditioned souls, like me, absorbed in the ego, thinking that we are the center and deserve to be served, instead of understanding we are small, tiny, insignificant fallible soldiers, dependent parts of something bigger. This is the yoga process: getting yourself out of the center so you can serve the center. Yet, in our illusion of grandeur, our misguided desires for happiness are similar to a fly banging repeatedly against a window in order to find an escape—only leaving that fly exhausted, dehydrated, flapping his legs and wings, lying on his back on the sill, waiting to be vacuumed up by the housecleaner. That's material existence.*

Mother Durga holds, in one of her many hands, a trident. This trident is designed to poke the embodied beings. Each prong represents one of the three miseries that make the embodied souls suffer.

Prong one: This represents pain caused by other beings. This could be a bee sting, getting punched in the nose by an aggressor, or an ex-spouse making you miserable.

Prong two: This represents the pain caused by the gods or the elements, as when it gets too cold or too hot, or when we get hit with tsunamis, tornados, earthquakes, etc. You get the picture.

Prong three: The third prong of the pitchfork is pain caused by one's own body or mind. It could be a migraine, a broken femur, and yes, even dysentery. A literal pain in the ass. Mixed with a mild fever.

Once we get a body, we're made to suffer by getting poked by any or all of these pokers. The yogis teach transcendence—not to fight against Durga or Nature. She is next level, out of our skill set. But we become dear to her Lord. By surrendering to Vishnu, he calls Durga, the wielder of the trident, and she backs off the embodied soul.

This happens when devotees connect with their spiritual self. Pain will always happen for one who is embodied. Nobody gets a pass from pain, but suffering is optional. When we identify with ourselves as spirit, and have the deep realization that the pain

> *we're experiencing is not us but in fact the body, it*
> *offers some type of respite. The agony subsides. The*
> *very evolve remain undisturbed and fearless.*

I was not evolved. Despite having supposedly learned that lesson in the toilet of the ashram, I was still attached to my body on the train to Kolkata, suffering in the thick heat of Madhya Pradesh, a state in central India. I was hot, uncomfortable, sweaty, slightly dizzy, and exhausted, since I couldn't sleep well on the train.

My mind suffered even more, jumping all over the place and creating drama that wasn't even present. I thought about the worst diseases that were common for Western travelers to catch in India: typhoid, malaria, cholera. Once, a monk told me that when he got malaria, it was so painful that he prayed he would die. I questioned why I was there in the first place. Couldn't God be found everywhere? Wasn't God in New York? If there was a God, was the only way to find Him to go to an isolated town nine thousand miles away with disorganized sewage disposal? What kind of God would make us do that? I started to worry about snake bites. Bed bugs. Indian prisons. Being trapped by a brainwashed cult in an isolated region and not being able to phone home. Drowning or getting swept away in a sacred river. I went from one extreme scenario to the next. Whatever pain I was feeling in my body paled in comparison to the suffering in my mind.

Then I realized that most of the pain in my life came not from the physical world but from the mental world. I spun my pain and discomfort out of control, almost forgetting why I was there and letting it influence my plans. This was silly. Yoga practices existed to help our minds become more peaceful. When the mind was at peace and anxiety and stress melted away, we could analyze our mind, and even change our mind. Then we could step out of that painful mental condition and see ourselves as the Analyzer, the Viewer, and the Spirit who has a mind that's fickle and subject to fear, stress, and being overwhelmed, but who was not us.

Reflecting on Vedic teachings provided some relief and hope for my future, but I was still a mess. I told myself this whole thing was an experiment to see if becoming a transcendentalist was real. I didn't want to feel that I'd over-committed to some vow or a lifestyle that I couldn't sustain. I needed to take this one step at a time. One day at a time.

The rhythmic pounding of wheels on steel was loud and strangely sooth-ing. I stopped mentally complaining and found some peace. When the train stopped at the next station, an elderly man came in, elegantly dressed in robes. He introduced himself as R. K. Goswami. He looked refined in his character and disposition and wore the traditional bhadra vesha, or auspi-cious clothing of old Indian men. His dhoti was white silk, somehow clean and wrinkle-free. My dhoti always looked like a mess. It was ready to fall off at any moment. The pleats were never even. I was too short for dhotis. They dragged. They didn't hang well. They often drooped from behind, leaving them stained with mud on the ends. Sometimes, they were too puffy and bulging around the crotch and belly, making me appear much fatter than I was. I didn't wear a dhoti naturally. This man on the train did. He wore it like he was born in it.

He sat down next to me. His beard was identical to Santa Claus's, and he wore a short-sleeved silk kurta, and a matching chadar thrown over his right shoulder completed the outfit. He was carrying a cheap Indian bag with a few items and wore rubber slippers. He couldn't have been a wandering beggar or a millionaire.

The gentleman took an interest in me immediately, probably because of the way I was dressed. The other monks were sleeping.

"What is your name, my dear?"

"Ray," I said, smiling and running my fingers through my mala.

"You like japa yoga," he said.

"Ah yes. It's my practice to remember God."

"Yes, it is a very good practice. My wife also practices. She also writes the holy name."

"Writes?"

"Yes. Every day for many years she writes for one hour the holy name in a book repeatedly. It is similar to japa but with a pen and paper. She has many, many notebooks filled with sacred words. It's another way to remember God."

R. K. Goswami came off as a sincere spiritualist and an elder, so I shut up and listened to him speak. I don't know how old he was, but his face was timeless and charming. Perfect teeth. He could have been in a toothpaste commercial.

"Let me tell you how to ruin your spiritual life, my dear." That caught me off guard. "Would you like to know? I will tell you so you can do the opposite."

"Yes, please," I said.

"All of your chanting, your spiritual practice, your meditation, bhajan and kirtan, your service to others, are all like investments into a godly account. Like depositing gold coins. These activities change you. They change your heart. Your mind. In one way, it is you and your work. But another way, it is the grace of Bhagavan. Bhagavan is lifting you higher and higher. Your storehouse of gems in your account is growing with each divine name flowing from your lips. But be careful of the thief. You can lose everything instantly."

"Who, or what, is the thief?" He was speaking in riddles now, so I edged closer.

"Sometimes we bring our bad habits from our previous life into our sacred life. You now have a sacred life, and you must not let the bad habits of your previous life come in. Keep them at the door. There are many thieves who want to plunder your wealth."

"Like who?"

"Some are big thieves. Expert thieves. Rogues. Scoundrels. Gundas. Some puny pickpockets. Their names are Kama, Krodha, Lobha, Moha. These are the plunderers. Lust, anger, greed, delusion."

At this point, I fully shut up and let him school me. I was enjoying his company and his playful analogy.

"Lust, or desire, manifests like a mirage in the desert," he said. "My home is in Rajasthan, and sometimes the cows will see water in the desert plains. It is not real water. It is not what it appears to be. It is a reflection of the heat on sand caused by the sun, but the cows walk to drink it. Then, just as they get closer, the mirage moves farther away, so they wander deeper into the desert. This continues, and they are found by their owners dead from exhaustion and dehydration. Our desires, kama, are the same. Our lower passions encourage us to enjoy this material world through our senses. Bollywood, your Hollywood, is inviting us for many romantic escapades. How will those escapades play out? It is already playing out in your country. No one is happy. Divorce is rampant. Children are abandoned. Tricked by kama. Like a mouse taking cheese from a baited trap."

He quoted the *Bhagavad Gita*, and I recognized the Sanskrit:

> A person who is not disturbed by the incessant flow
> of desires that enter like rivers into the ocean, which
> is ever being filled but is always still, can alone achieve
> peace and not the man who strives to satisfy such desires.

Then he continued to tell the story.

"When our kama is frustrated, we develop krodha, or anger. We either want something and don't get it, or we want something and it doesn't fulfill us, and then this krodha arises. This anger remains in our heart. But, like the cow, when you do get to the watering hole, it moves back even more. Material life becomes sad. Then lobha. Strong attachment to things that will not even satisfy us. Degrading our consciousness. From there, moha. We become completely bewildered. The materialist is bewildered like a madman."

I nod, remembering some of my activities as a madman.

"I'm sure you have friends who think you are mad for giving up this maya. In the insane asylum, my dear, the sane seem crazy."

"I have two questions, Pandit-ji," I said, addressing him with a term of reverence. Out of all of these plunderers who steal your spiritual wealth, which is the worst?"

"The worst plunderer of your spiritual wealth? The *very* worst? That is easy. Criticism of saintly people. Or criticizing anyone. Everyone carries the Lord in their heart. Do you understand this? People can do so much tapas—spiritual discipline—but the greatest tapas is to control your tongue from finding fault with others. May I tell you a story?"

"Of course!" I said, sadly realizing that I was a black belt in finding fault and criticism.

"There once was a king who was sponsoring a feast for all the Brahmins in his kingdom. All the priests were so grateful, and the king appreciated them so. He had his own cooks prepare this wonderful feast and fed all the priests and their families with delicious vegetable preparations, puris, milk sweets, and fancy rice. At that time an eagle was flying overhead with a dead cobra in its talons. A drop of the venom fell from the mouth of the cobra and landed on the plate of one of the Brahmins. The Brahmin ate the next bite of the poisoned rice and fell dead into his prasad. Now, the killing of a Brahmin is a very serious offense to the Lord," said R. K. Goswami in a foreboding tone. "Do you know who Yamaraja is? He is the god of yama, or control. He and his assistants observe what people have done in this lifetime and give them the appropriate karma for their behavior. Yamaraja looked at his assistants and said, 'This Brahmin is dead. Who should receive the karma for this?'"

I could tell he enjoyed sharing this story, and I enjoyed listening to him, like a young child and a grandfather.

"One of the assistants of Yamaraja spoke up," said R. K. Goswami. "'Definitely the king!' he said.

"'The king?' Yamaraja replied, 'But why? He was merely honoring these Brahmins. His intention was to give affection. Not death.'

"Another spoke up. 'Definitely it should be the snake! His mouth was filled with venom. It's the venom that killed the Brahmin.'

"Yamaraja spoke again. 'We cannot give karma to the snake. The snake was dead. How can he get karma for something he didn't do?'

"'The eagle?' said another assistant of Yamaraja. 'The eagle is the one that killed the snake and was flying over the Brahmin community.'

"They were all puzzled, and Yamaraja, being thoughtful, said, 'Let us wait and think about this before we distribute the appropriate reactions to the appropriate party.'

"Weeks passed and some pilgrims were coming to visit the kingdom because it housed an ancient and beautiful temple of Lord Ramachandra. As they were approaching the kingdom, the road forked, and an older woman was sitting between the roads under a tree, shading herself from the noon sun.

"'O mother,' the pilgrims addressed her, 'we are looking for a temple of Lord Rama in a nearby kingdom. Which is the direction that we should go?'

"The old lady replied flippantly. 'You mean the kingdom where the king kills Brahmins? Is that the kingdom you're looking for?' she asked cynically. 'It is to your left.' And she pointed in the direction of the kingdom where the unfortunate incident had happened. At that time, Yamaraja and his servants knew who to give the karma to. He gave all the karma of the dead Brahmin to the old lady."

"Why?" I asked. "I don't get it. What did she have to do with the incident?"

"The lesson is that if you criticize somebody who is innocent of a crime, you receive the karma for the crime. As the faultfinder who is relishing that soul's misfortune, you have now become intimately implicated in that karma. Only Yamaraja can judge. It is not our position. When we become the judge, we poison ourselves with hatred and become polluted and thus suffer the consequences. Our position is to love, not to condemn. One who judges indiscriminately suffers in a pool of hatred."

I sat quietly, reflecting on my own gossipy, sarcastic past. I swallowed and said, "But what if that person *did* do the crime and you just call them out on it? What if they *did* do the wrong action? What's wrong with saying that? Isn't that reasonable? They've done something. Call them out."

"If the person did the crime and you criticize them for it, or 'call them out' as you put it, the faultfinder will get partial karma for the perpetrators' crimes."

"Why!" I spoke loudly and almost defensively, thinking how many times I'd called people out on wrong actions.

"Because they are relishing a person's poor choices," said R. K. Goswami. "They are thinking themself superior to the culprit, and they are not. They themselves are just a moment away from a poor action. Every person is carrying God within their hearts, my dear. Yama is the judge of how they should be rectified. This is how problematic criticism is. It destroys people's lives. You must always be careful about what comes out of your mouth. Since Bhagavan is all-loving, he cannot tolerate insults to those he loves. In the same way, it hurts a parent when someone offends their child. We are all children of God. We implicate ourselves in this samsara with our vile gossip, steeped in our own arrogance or speculation, desperately trying to make ourselves seem justified or righteous. Criticism is the greatest thief of your spiritual wealth."

R. K. Goswami got up. "This is my stop," he said. He gathered his things and looked at me seriously. "My dear, if you will add something to your life, just do this one thing: Give up the desire to find fault with others and try to find their good instead." He broke eye contact with me and got off the train.

* * *

The Howrah railway station in West Bengal was considered the biggest train station in the world, serving six hundred passenger trains and over one million travelers. I stepped off the train into a cacophony of sounds and sweat, carefully following Mohan and the four monks I was traveling with. Shaken up and a little exhausted, I dodged beggars, businessmen, and families as we made our way through the crowded platform. I tried to stay focused, as the scene was overwhelming and I was slightly fearful I'd lose them. A van picked us up and brought me to the Kolkata Krishna Bhakti temple, where I'd be staying for a few days.

I was introduced to Keshava Das, an older Indian man who spoke fluent English. He was round-bodied and sweet, with a big smile on his face. Some of the monks in Vrindavan asked him to take care of me, so he invited me to stay in his room with a few others living on the floor. That was luxury compared to where the rest of the monks were staying: on the roof under mosquito nets or in the men's ashram. He was not a monk but lived like one. His wife was presently with his mother. He was jovial and bright-eyed. He told me he went to university in the United States to learn restaurant management, and met his guru, A. C. Bhaktivedanta Swami, there in the 1970s. After he met his guru, he wanted to give his life to the ashram and the devotees.

He put his arm around me. "Oh, Ray," he said, "you know what I miss the most about the US?" I was under the impression that he was going to say something deeply spiritual, but his answer was Philadelphia brand cream cheese. "I loved that!" he said. "Oh my God, I cannot get that here, and I miss it!" I laughed and could relate, as I was missing foods, too.

"Do you know what I miss?" I asked.

"What?"

"Peanut butter. I haven't had it in months. I would eat it at home every day."

"I know where I can get you some, Bhakta Ray. I know a place! We can go tomorrow afternoon. Get a good night's sleep, and I'll see you in the morning for the temple program."

I woke up early and went to the morning program at 4:30 a.m. There was always something magical about being up and singing that early in the morning, with the tinkling of the morning bells of the priest and the wafting of incense.

During the japa time, I went up to the roof, where many of the brahma-charis had slept and from where I could see Kolkata. The city seemed to be filled with religious people. I could hear the arati bells ringing in other houses and see people doing their puja to Krishna or Durga. I had heard that Kolkata was quite beautiful during the British raj and that it was called the crest jewel of India. That day I wandered the streets. There were lovely British-looking parks, square city blocks, and square sacred ponds fed by the holy Ganges. I saw modern businesswomen power walking around the ponds, and it was almost as though I was back in New York City. But then next to a businesswoman would be a sadhu living under a banyan tree and worshiping a Shiva deity that fit snuggly into a crevice of the oddly shaped tree.

Banyan trees have smooth bark and branches that drop roots, which then grow more trees, creating an ever-expanding tree that drops, sprouts, and takes over. Some become massive and make tiny homes for mendicants. I watched the sadhu with long, matted hair get up and, just wearing a G-string, walk into the pond as if he was from another age and taking his bath in a sacred lake or river. It was as though a modern city was built on top of an ancient village. I suppose it was. The British created this city from three villages, one of which was Kolkata, or the place of Kali, as Kali worship was very popular in that area.

While walking back to the temple, I drank a coconut sold by a man who climbed a tree to get it. I carefully dodged taxis and hand-pulled rickshaws in this land where street rules barely existed.

In Kolkata, I was a little like a dog off the leash. There was a lot of accountability in Vrindavan, and our spiritual practice was joyful but serious. It was not a vacation place. It was a holy place with little to no tourists. Most people there were serious practitioners of the Vedic path, and I had older monks checking up on me. Here, I was a tourist and Kolkata was a major city with major maya. My mind wandered around the streets. Everything seemed intriguing. I still was not completely comfortable wearing my dhoti. I fidgeted. My robe knot cut into the tender flesh on my hip, and I hadn't quite gotten the hang of Brahmin underwear and feared I never would. They would unhinge and leave me hanging, so to speak.

Keep focused on the mantra! I would tell myself when I was on a japa walk. *Hare Krishna, Hare Krishna . . .*

If I wanted to, I could disappear into the Kolkata streets with no accountability. I found myself looking at beautiful women, then hating myself for it, as I was dressed like a monk. I also looked at all the delicious food I wanted to eat, which was not sanctified like it was in the temple. I was mesmerized by the shops, restaurants, and Bollywood movies. The metaphysical—yet not necessarily spiritual—things drew me in. Palm readers, psychics, mystics. It was difficult to maintain a monk's mindset ("How can I serve?") over a tourist's mindset ("How can I enjoy?"). I remembered the teachings of both Satyaraja in New York and Swami-ji in Vrindavan: *Do I want to* be *God or* serve *God?* I realized how Vrindavan's potent environment kept me focused and strong. I thought it was my own deep spiritual connection. It wasn't. It was being in that sacred place with sacred people that kept my consciousness high.

What was I doing in Kolkata? I felt like such a fake. A hypocrite. I never knew controlling my senses would be so difficult. And it wasn't like the world thought I was a better man for it. My friends and family thought I was nuts. I was trying to be the absolute best version of myself, and everyone thought I had lost my mind or had been indoctrinated by a dangerous cult. That was tough.

But I stood firm in my conviction that sense control and developing spiritual vision were the best things I could do for humanity. To develop love over lust, giving over greed, and simplicity over complication was a noble act and that's why I had chosen to move forward despite public opinion. That didn't mean it wasn't arduous. But I'd thought I would have been much more advanced in my spiritual practice by that point.

When I got back to the temple, I noticed a beautiful holy man in his seventies or eighties wearing a dhoti, with sacred markings on his forehead. He had a long snow-white beard and greased-backed white hair. He was holding the hand of a young girl not more than eight. They went to the altar. The little girl, like the old man, put her hands in namaste, bowed down, and stood back up again, ardently looking at the deities. Then they both stepped to the side of the altar, went to a large basket of discarded garlands and prasad flowers, and draped them around their necks. My heart melted. Perhaps this was the young girl's grandfather. How sweet. What a gift to give your grandchild. A heart filled with devotion.

I noticed this ritual three days in a row. Same old man leading this young girl into the temple, bowing, praying, getting the old garlands and wearing them home.

Keshava Das saw me watching and smiled. "Fascinating, isn't it?"

"Yes! This holy man brings his granddaughter here every day? How sweet is that?"

Keshava Das laughed. No, Prabhu, this is not his granddaughter. He is not a sadhu. This little girl is from a very wealthy family. He is her servant. She makes him come every day. And they've been coming for years. They've been coming since she was very little. This child has had an intense attraction to Krishna and devotion to him since she was a toddler. The man will do whatever she tells him."

* * *

One night, Keshava Das told me to wake up early because he was going to take me on an adventure. That's all he said, and he wouldn't tolerate me prying about what it was. I was excited. I was up early. Keshava Das directed me downstairs to a car with a driver. The streets were empty.

Our car pulled up to banks of the Hooghly River, a branch of the sacred Ganges that flowed southwest through Kolkata.

"Every successful man in Kolkata comes here for a massage, a sugarcane juice, and a bath in the Ganges," Keshava Das said.

My face lit up. "Okay!"

There was a line of very expensive cars with drivers waiting. The sun still hadn't risen, so it was sort of eerie and cool. Kolkata was a major shipping port, so it reminded me of the docks of any major US city except that the river was sacred. Although you could hear cargo boats being loaded and unloaded, you could also hear sacred sounds, like men worshiping deities of Ganesh, Radha, and Krishna. A group of women in saris, singing prayers, walked into the sacred water fully clothed. The juxtaposition caught me off guard. The holy people seemed oblivious of the city that was built around and on top of them. They were in another world.

Wooden beds were laid out, and small men who were naked except for some cloth wrapped around them (as if they were wearing shorts) waved us over. They were there to massage us. I was ordered in a language I didn't understand to strip down to my underwear. Keshava Das did the same. The little men mounted me, covered me in mustard oil, and gripped, elbowed, and slapped me. It wasn't gentle. It was borderline painful. But these men were pros, and they took full control, using their hands, feet, and forearms to renew my body. They knew exactly where to apply pressure, where to squeeze, and where to occasionally slap. After forty minutes, it was over. Keshava Das paid them and took me over to the Ganges riverbank. There was a ship not far from us, and incense burned behind us. We shared the bank with pilgrims and dockworkers.

"This is the sacred Ganges," Keshava Das said.

I knew the river was considered a goddess who gives material enjoyment, freedom from suffering, and devotion to God. I had read that holy people since before recorded time had bathed in her waters. I had read that it was better to be an outcaste or a turtle living on her banks than to be a wealthy king living far from her. I had been waiting for this day but pictured a more romantic way to take my first bath in her waters. Although I understood the concept of sacred waters and the importance of bathing our body as if a baptism, I was slightly hesitant. It was sort of dirty, like a river flowing through New York City. There was some garbage around. I balked. I looked at Keshava Das.

"Prabhu, it's a little dirty, don't you think?"

He was somewhat shocked. And with a big, animated smile he said, "Bhakta Ray! Don't you understand where you are? This is Mother Ganges. She's flowing from the lotus feet of Lord Vishnu. No matter what is put into her waters, she cannot become contaminated. On the contrary, everything she touches becomes purified."

He was fully convinced that, despite the obvious messiness of the environment, this was a magical place, and the opportunity should not be wasted. I put my material reasoning on hold, and in his enthusiasm, I moved forward. We bowed down like a stick, offering our respect to Mother Ganges.

Keshava Das recited a prayer: "O Mother Ganges, take away my sorrows, my disease, difficulties, and wrong attitudes. You are the essence of the three worlds and a necklace around the earth. O goddess, you alone are my refuge in this world of birth and death."

It was beautiful. We grabbed palmfuls of water and offered them to the Ganges, ritualistically representing an offering of our love: cupping our hands, lifting the water, and letting it rain into the river. Then, with reverence, we walked into her waters. Keshava Das was enthusiastic. I was brave but stopped in my tracks when I realized that there was a bloated pig floating in the water. My jaw dropped. "Keshava Das!" I motioned toward the balloon of fur bobbing two meters away.

He gave me a head bobble and said, "Ganga Mayi ki jaya!" which meant "All glories to Mother Ganges!" and ignored my fear, submerging himself in the water. So did I.

"Don't you feel different?" he said, smiling. "No matter what you want in this world, Mother Ganges will supply it. Everybody in India knows this. Everyone comes to her. The sick, the distressed, the devoted, the mystics. Everyone." Then he went on to tell me how he knew a person who had a miracle cure from a skin disease by bathing in her waters. "Modern people say it's because there are so many medicinal herbs in the mountains that tributaries flow through that the water has something magical and healing properties to it. But that's not it. It's flowing from the higher worlds, Ray."

I nodded. *Why not?* I thought. The sun had started rising. I could see clearly.

We dried ourselves off, then put on our clothes and walked back past the massage table to a man with a big metal wheel and a bunch of sugar canes. He was selling sugarcane juice with ginger and lemon. A divine combination. Keshava Das put up two fingers, and the juice wallah started grinding long canes. Green juice rained into a silver pitcher.

"A magical elixir," Keshava Das said. "One of the healthiest foods you could drink, according to Ayurveda."

I had never had anything like it. *This is normal life*, I thought. Bathing in sacred waters, taking care of your body with massage, rising early, and drinking freshly squeezed juices in the morning.

I liked Kolkata and the ashram and the devotees.

*   *   *

The next morning, I went on my normal japa walk through the streets. I tried to meditate on the sacred syllables but again found my mind

FROM PUNK TO MONK

wandering. It was about 5:30 a.m., and the sun was still not fully up. I saw an elderly man dressed in a dhoti and a shawl in the distance. He had the thick clay markings of Vaishnava tilak on his forehead, slightly thicker than the kind I wore on mine. His represented a lineage from South India.

I was taken aback when I saw him squat down, lift his dhoti, and defecate in the gutter on the side of the street. I had studied a book in Vrindavan on the etiquette of Vaishnavas, the followers of Vaishnavism. The manual was several hundred years old. It dealt with nuanced dos and don'ts for people practicing bhakti yoga: *Don't point your feet at somebody while you're sitting. Don't step over somebody. Don't eat with your left hand. Wash your hands if you touch your mouth. Don't place sacred literature on the floor, as it represents Saraswati, the goddess of learning. Don't bring your mala into the toilet.*

One rule that stood out at the time and came to mind now was "A Vaishnava should never defecate in the street." *Who would ever defecate in the street?* I thought when I read it. Perhaps it was written for people in another age, when low-class people did such things. But now I watched a man dressed like a Vaishnava, a worshiper of Vishnu, squatting down and doing just that. *How dare he!* I thought. *Doesn't he know the etiquette?*

Later that day, I met up with Keshava Das. It was a holiday for one of the saints in our tradition, so we followed an observance of fasting until noon, then having an honorific feast at 12:30. It was delicious, with vegetable preparations I had never tasted before, fancy rice with saffron and turmeric, making it appear yellow, and puris. When it was all done, a server came around with a little leaf cup and dumped two balls in a syrup into it.

"What are these?" I asked Keshava Das, who was sitting next to me.

"You like sweets, and you've never had gulab jamun?!" he said "Oh! Bhakta Ray, wait till you taste this. But you better love sweets to appreciate it!"

"I do! I do!" I popped one of the spongy balls dripping with sugary rose and cardamon syrup into my mouth, and my taste buds exploded. It was the best food I had ever had.

"Bring Bhakta Ray more gulab jamun!" Keshava Das said.

The server put four more on my plate. I ate them quickly. "So delicious!" I sipped from the cup, finishing all the syrup.

"Eat more!" said Keshava Das. "Our cook who makes this is the best!"

More gulab jamun were dumped into my leaf cup, and I ate them. I didn't stop until I ate fourteen gulab jamun. Then I lay down on my left side in a sugar high, smiling like a drunkard, mumbling to myself, "What a feast, what a feast, what a feast!"

Keshava Das saw me belly-filled and resting in the same place where I had been eating. "Bhakta Ray, today I want you to go out with the monks," he said. "There's a big metaphysical book fair going on in the park near the Ganges. I want you to go and help the brahmacharis distribute sacred books. So many different yoga societies will set up book tables, but hardly anybody is teaching bhakti. Go there today and help our boys. You'll be good at it."

We drove into town in two minivans loaded with books, dioramas, tables, tablecloths, and some little packages of prasad laddus, or sweet balls, to distribute to the public. It almost seemed like Central Park in New York City. People were picnicking, playing with children, and leisurely walking. Yoga societies were setting up book tables promoting their particular ashram and guru lineages as we set up ours. It was a beautiful day, and right across the main road I could see the beautiful Ganges River flowing.

Then my stomach made a noise—a noise I had never heard my stomach make. Like a squealing sound. As it squealed, it violently jerked back and forth in a way it had never moved before. My insides were doing something weird. I remembered the fourteen gulab jamun I ate. I guess I shouldn't have eaten fourteen without expecting some type of reaction. I quicky grabbed one of the older monks. "Excuse me, is there some type of porta-potty out here? Some bathroom, public restroom, or something I could use?" I asked desperately.

The monk looked at me confused, shaking his head. "No, Prabhu, there is no porta-potty, I am not knowing what you mean."

"Well, when do we go back to the ashram?" I asked.

"Five hours." He continued to set up his book table.

My stomach made another squealing sound, which propelled my insides to shift, contract, and pulse rapidly.

"Five hours! I need a porta-potty now!"

I didn't know where I was going, but I started to run—desperately run—looking for any place that could serve as a bathroom. The more I ran through the park in my flowing robes and flip-flops, the more pathetic and hopeless I felt. It was a Sunday afternoon, complete with family outings, people on bicycles, kids kicking balls, and some teens playing cricket. Here I was, some white kid dressed in Hindu attire, with a soured face and one hand on my stomach, sprinting to nowhere. I couldn't take it any longer. While still running I attempted to loosen my knotted robe for relief as it was putting pressure on my abdomen. Instead of loosening it, it untied itself completely and fell to the ground around my ankles, leaving me streaking and tripping across the park. I was wearing nothing under my robes except my Brahmin underwear. Humiliated, I surrendered to my body and shamefully defecated in public—just like the elderly man I had criticized for defecating in the street.

Instant karma! I thought. I finally learned the lesson of not judging others too harshly. We are all moments away from performing the same vile activity we condemn. As I squatted in that park, my dhoti partially covering my embarrassment, I reflected on that old man, my arrogance, and how far I had to go on my spiritual journey. I felt hideous inside and out, especially as flies started to overwhelm me. I pulled myself together, covered my private parts, ran across the street, and dove in the Ganges to cleanse myself internally and externally.

* * *

I took a few days to visit the sacred land of Mayapur, which was four hours north of Kolkata through jungles, mango trees, and tropical farms. I didn't really get to know anybody there, so my exploring was all done privately. Mayapur was the birthplace of Sri Chaitanya Mahaprabhu, the Kirtan Avatar. It was beautiful and on the bank of the Ganges River, down a poorly paved road lined with ashram after ashram of Radha Krishna temples. On the third day, I went to the boatman, who for less than a rupee shuttled me across the river, which was as wide as the Hudson. It was a motorless boat. The boatman only had oars and a stick. He spoke no English, and as I crossed that majestic river surrounded by date and coconut palms, temple spires, and simple village life, it seemed as though I could have time-traveled. On the other side of the river was Nabadwip, another holy spot and ancient center of learning. Popular here was also the worship of Kali. I crossed the river that day unknowingly stumbling into Kali Puja, or the festival of Mother Kali. There were big floats of the goddess set up with flowers, incense, and burning lamps. Teens were playing drums. Many people were leading goats with ropes around their necks against their will, causing them to call out. I didn't quite understand what was going on with all the goats until my eyes fell upon a man with a knife slitting a goat's throat as an offering to Mother Kali.

As a vegetarian, I was disturbed and quickly realized I wanted nothing more to do with this festival. I found my way back to my Krishna temple and devotees who rallied behind the theory of ahimsa, or nonviolence. No goat killing for me. I got back to the boatman and headed back to the Mayapur guesthouse I was staying in. I started to think about my next plan of action for my life.

I'd learned deep life lessons in India, and although I felt like I was on the right path, I had loud callings to wrap up unfinished business at home and say goodbye to India for now. It served the purpose of rooting me and directing me, for giving faith in the process and context for the tradition.

But there were details of my life I had to figure out. I knew I needed an official goodbye to my fans. I'd left abruptly at our band's height. Perhaps a final musical release. Writing and recording records were sonic diaries for me. I needed to write a record and put this journal to rhyme and music. I needed to see my mother to see how she was faring after losing my father. Then I needed to figure out what was my unique offering. What was my devotional service or contribution to the world? Perhaps I needed to find a community or an ashram in the States. I was definitely at some type of crossroads, but at this point I filled my cup by wandering around India like a young sadhu.

I went back to Kolkata, stayed in the ashram, explored the city and the Gariahat Market, continued journaling, and bathed in the Ganges one more time, promising and praying that I could return soon. I decided to make it back to see my family at Christmas.

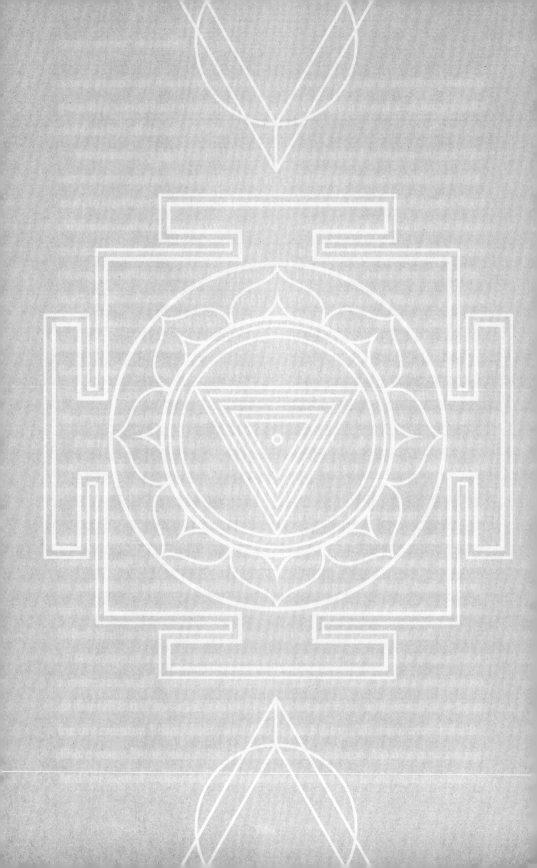

CHAPTER 8

A RETURN TO MUSIC

I made it to my mother's house in Connecticut just in time for Christmas Eve day. I had come late the night before and hadn't seen her or any of my siblings. I just fell asleep in one of the guest rooms. I rose early and started my chanting meditation in the kitchen at 4 a.m. I had no jet lag. I had written my mother several times from India, but she had no idea what I was doing there. That all changed when she walked into the kitchen at about 5:30 a.m. I was wearing my orange robes, had a monk's shaved head with a ponytail and an orange wrap around my bare chest. I had my clay markings on my forehead, arms, and shoulders, which were clearly visible. She stared at me in disbelief.

"I thought you said you were becoming a priest!" Her face puckered.

"I *am* a priest," I said. Being a monk was practically the same thing.

"A *Christian* priest!"

"I *am* a Christian priest, Mom. There's one God. We're all trying to love. You, me, Jesus. Everybody wants connection to God. It's all the same, Mom. And I'm sure if Christ was here right now, he'd high-five me."

She wasn't convinced. "But what about the robes?" she said. "Why?"

"What do you think Christ wore? Levi's?

My mother was soon pacified when she realized I hadn't lost my mind. I decided to stay with her that month, as all my siblings went back to their respective homes around the country. It was just me and her in the big colonial house where I grew up.

I made a commitment to write my farewell musical offering to my fans—a record to be finished and recorded in thirty days. I moved into my old room in the attic. I did my morning meditation up there privately. I fasted till noon every day, and then I picked up a guitar and started writing what I thought would be my swan song, my final recording. I was convinced that music and the music scene were the cause of a lot of my internal turmoil. Little did I know, a few years later the *Bhagavad Gita* would flip that story as I delved further into its wisdom. The *Gita* was not an ordinary book about giving up one's life and going AWOL to find God. It was about applying your talents with a spiritual focus. It just hadn't fully sunk in at that point. I thought, immaturely, that to be spiritual you must give up your passions—after all, didn't desire cause my suffering in the first place?

At noon, I'd come downstairs and make my mom rice, beans, tofu, and tahini. I would offer it on a little altar of Krishna that I kept in the kitchen next to a picture of Jesus, and sit and eat with her. In the evening I did a little meditation on the holy places I visited. Before my head hit the pillow, I would privately sing some of the devotional songs I learned in the ashram. I kept sleeping on the floor to remind me of ashram life. Sometimes, I'd have to take a break and walk out into the cold of a Connecticut January to get my head clear. I found that with marathon sessions of writing music and lyrics, I sometimes had to step away and change environments. Going outside into nature helped.

I had journals of lyrics, poems, and realizations that I had jotted down while I was traveling in India. Topics included the futility of material existence, the randomness of life and death, the urgency to find our spiritual calling, and how we can become addicted to laziness and comfort. After twenty-eight days straight, I called some friends who were accomplished musicians, and after two days of practicing and showing them how the songs went, we went into the studio to record. Quickest record I ever did.

They asked me what I wanted to title it. I looked at my journal. Some pages were just scribbles of phrases, words, statements, proclamations. One word that appeared repeatedly was *shelter*. I nodded. That was it. *What we're all looking for*, I thought.

*   *   *

Porcell heard I was at my mother's and working on music. He called the home phone. He was in a new straight-edge band called Judge that had become very popular. He asked me if I would consider doing a three-month European tour with Youth of Today, just this one time. A bubble of material excitement started to rise in my heart.

Europe was always a magical place in my mind. It holds an old-world charm for many in the United States, for its cafés, architecture, hilltop castles, massive cathedrals, stone buildings, cobblestone streets, and, of course, the art and culture. The United States, as we know it, is a relatively new country. Nothing appears old or ancient. Native American cultures have been plowed under and paved over, shopping malls built over their holy places.

My spiritual intelligence knew this was a deep-rooted material desire and that it wouldn't fulfill me, but for the next two weeks, it kept tapping me on the shoulder until I finally conceded. I'd go to Europe on tour while keeping my vows, my focus, my celibacy, and my study.

*   *   *

I quickly realized this tour was going to be difficult. I had already tasted the sweetness of raising the bar high with my consciousness, meditation, chanting, and disciplined living; now, due to a desire to see Europe, I was back on the road with the dudes. My old friends. I loved these guys like brothers, but I had grown into a new man, now at age twenty-three. I felt like I'd gotten a glimpse into another world. My adventures into spiritual life, walking barefoot with sadhus, bathing in sacred rivers, sitting in meditative stillness before the sun rose, and dancing in kirtan with pure joy gave me an internal high I'd never experienced before. This world of touring around nightclubs that stunk of beer and smoke with their bathroom graffiti of penises—it all seemed abhorrent now.

In 1989, the clean-cut, straight-edge, hardcore scene that we championed was as developed in Europe as it was in the United States, so a lot of our performances were at squats— often abandoned big buildings filled with anarchist homeless kids, either loosely permitted by the government or not. The squatters' theory was one of entitlement: *There's a building. We need a place to live. It's abandoned. We're moving in.* In the United States there was more pushback against squatters and squatters' rights. In Europe, the squatters were incredibly organized. They often had electricity and running water. It was sort of a postapocalyptic society, communally cooking, hosting art or music performances, and growing community gardens. Some were quite impressive. Some were downright disgusting. As straight-edge practitioners, we liked our punk rock clean, organized, and sanitary. I didn't realize what I was signing up for when we took this tour. When audiences heard we didn't drink, they whipped beer at us, which was humiliating, disgusting, and—when contained in half-liter bottles— downright dangerous. This type of treatment triggered my ego's retaliation and anger, and thus I suffered.

One night I sat backstage at a massive abandoned theater in Copenhagen, one of the more disgusting squats we performed in. I leaned against the wall, thinking, *Why did I give up the ashram? For this?* There were corked bottles of urine lining the walls, which along with rocks and bricks, squatters dropped on cops who tried to trespass. The squatters had created a fortress out of the theater. Night after night the situation was similar. The shows were big and sold out, but the energy was dark and negative compared with our US audiences. At that point each city had only a handful of dedicated Youth of Today fans (our fame increased after we officially disbanded).

It felt like it was a drunken punk party, and we were the hired entertainment. Our message of peace, unity, self-control, and positive living seemed to fall on deaf ears. Often, I felt like I was performing the soundtrack for hell, where people lay intoxicated on the ground with ripped clothes, leather jackets, spiked hair, and jailhouse tattoos. Sitting in that decrepit, poorly lit building, looking at the graffiti on the walls, witnessing people walk around like drunk zombies, I thought, *If there is a hell, it must be something like this.*

I'd get inspiration from walking and chanting around the cities before the performances. This was my only solace. The beautiful streets of Stockholm, Brussels, Amsterdam, and Florence were all breathtaking. I went into the massive Duomo di Milano, the biggest cathedral in Italy and the third biggest in the world. After marveling at the architecture and the devotion it took to build it—it was started in 1386 and took almost six hundred years to complete—I entered, touched the holy water with my right hand and performed the sign of the cross, touching my forehead, sternum, and left and right shoulders, as I did growing up in the Catholic Church. I didn't know exactly what it meant but performed the sacred ritual anyway.

The cathedral served as both a place of prayer and a museum of sorts, where guides took school children or tourists. Old religious Italian ladies lit candles, kneeled, and prayed. This was a bit unique, as many of the other European cathedrals that gave me peace and stillness during my travels were merely museums. It seemed like people had lost faith in God and invested their faith in consumption.

I sat in a pew, then kneeled and began to pray audibly, but softly, in English.

"Lord, I don't know why I have come to this planet in this incarnation as Ray Cappo. I know I have something to contribute to this world. Although I'm charmed by Europe, the cities, the architecture, the cafés . . . it's *really* charming. Please don't let me get lost in the charm. Please protect me from this maya. It's like an ornately wrapped Christmas present with nothing inside. I know it's the same illusions going on here as back home! Just a different charming package! People are lost. Confused. Eating. Working. Feeling busy. But in their hearts they're busy doing nothing. Sleeping. Pursuing sexual partners. At best a family. Exactly like in America. Exactly like the entire world. Exactly like animals. I know there's a reason why we're here. I know there's more to this world, and I'm refusing to let the romance of these charming places intoxicate me. Please, help me keep my vows of celibacy and meditation. Please, help me control my speech, which wants to lash out and criticize. Please, help me keep this internal process where I should change instead of yelling at the world to change. Please, help me be tolerant of the other guys in the band instead of trying to preach to them. Please, Lord, help me learn to love those who are different from me, even if they're not on my path."

I already knew from my time in Kolkata that sense control was easier in the confines of the ashram, but Europe tested me further. Wandering through Europe without the association of monks had me looking around like a kid in a candy store with a credit card. I could indulge in anything with no accountability. I was also free to face the consequences of such indulgence. In Western religion, God was made out to be a wicked, heartless sadist who laid down all these rules on us, waiting for us to slip up so we could be punished in this life or the next. This was not the Vedic perspective. God was love. God was a loving force. Rules were merely there for our benefit to protect us from pain.

I frequently sat, chanted, prayed, and reflected in European churches. Who would have thought six hundred years ago that a young man would come in here and chant the *Mahamantra*? That being said, I considered myself on Jesus's team more than ever. Just with a twist of Eastern thought. The architecture of these cathedrals was awe inspiring, and I appreciated the feeling of sacredness and holiness when I entered them. But they were also dark and dreary, if not a little sad, compared to Indian temples, which were fun and festive. In my experience Indian temples were also more kid-friendly. I reflected on my parents, who bribed me with Dunkin' Donuts to go to church. In retrospect, I appreciated their effort. I often took the bait they offered.

* * *

While in Copenhagen, I went in search of a Krishna temple but ended up at a Buddhist monastery. The priest was dressed in maroon robes with a golden undergarment. The monastery was tastefully decorated and smelled of incense. I engaged in a lively discussion with the priest.

"This entire world is an illusion," he said. "A mirage."

"I agree," I said, nodding. "It appears as one thing and then leads us into pain. Is pain a mirage? An illusion also?"

"Yes, it is created in the mind," he said. "There is no pain. It is an illusion as well. We are constantly giving meaning to experiences. It is the meaning that causes us to suffer and enjoy."

That was profound. I thought of the drunk punk squatters. Many people would think they were disgusting. *They* thought they were having the time of their lives. According to their values, different people put different meaning on the same experience.

"What about happiness?" I asked

"It is also an illusion. Also created in the mind. We are meaning makers, Ray. Our minds merely create meaning where there is no meaning. Things happen and then we ascribe meaning to them. The meaning we ascribe is according to our own past experiences and conditioning. Some people see the ocean, and they think the ocean is pleasurable. Some people see the ocean, and they have great fear.

"We are meaning makers!" I repeated.

"Yes, exactly."

"So, what about God? A creator? A lover? A friend? What's your conception of God?"

"We are meaning makers," he repeated. "We are merely fabricating God. Giving meaning where there is no meaning. There is no personal deity, Ray."

"But how do you know? How do you know to say there isn't some supreme intelligence, designer, maintainer? How do you know it's not just our own arrogance saying, 'Nothing is bigger or greater than me'?"

He didn't answer right away. "The truth is that there is nothing," he finally said, louder.

"Nothing?" I asked.

"Nothing."

"So, you really believe that the absolute truth, the source of everything, the gods, the goddesses that you have painted on the walls in this temple, love, music, beauty, death, mountains, oceans, penguins, everything . . . is just *nothing*?"

"Ultimately it is all nothing. Even your illusion is nothing."

"So if I were to kill you, or love you, both are nothing?"

He nodded in affirmation.

"Then why," I pleaded, "are you, the monks, the bodhisattvas, working so hard in meditation, chanting, using deities, gongs, rising early, restricting the diet if it's all nothing? Why all the discipline if it all means nothing anyway?"

"Because we do not *know* it is nothing."

It was a poor response in my humble opinion. "If it's nothing, why do anything? Why even talk to me? It's nothing. Do you really know what nothing means?" I was getting a little upset. I refused to believe that torturing kittens and kissing babies were the same—that they were both nothing.

I liked many Buddhist scriptures, but after this conversation, I was confused. I'm not saying that he represented all Buddhists, either. I don't know if he was advanced in the teachings or the explanations or not, but I left skeptical and frustrated. I did not want to live in this nihilistic world where everything was nothing. Perhaps, even the thought that it was nothing was nothing. So, why not reject it here and now? The Buddha taught compassion. Why be compassionate if it's all nothing? He taught nonviolence. Why be nonviolent if it makes no difference in a nothing world? Why not do whatever the hell you want to do? In a world of nothing, there is no wrong or right, good or bad, hate or love. I found no place for a peaceful mind to land or anything practical in his line of reasoning. Disturbed, I walked back to meet the band. I knew there was something. After all, even nothing must have a source.

* * *

I was excited to return to London and hoped to visit people I had met last time on my layover to India, including the temple monks who took such good care of me, Poly Styrene, and Jonathan and Maria. Both Poly Styrene and Jonathan came to our performance at the School of Oriental and African Studies. I was honored that Poly came, and she invited the band to stay over with her and her husband that night.

When I saw Jonathan, I immediately embraced him, and he joyfully returned the embrace. Although we only had a short time together in London, I connected deeply with both him and his wife, Maria. I was a little surprised that Jonathan was alone. When I first met him, he and Maria were inseparable.

"Where is Maria?" I asked, smiling.

His face changed from smiling to slightly smiling, but it was obvious his mind was deep in thought, as if I'd stumped him on *Jeopardy*. "Maria is gone," he said soberly. "She died. I'm so sad to say."

I was taken aback—I had met them not even a year before. They were healthy and vibrant, with great attitudes. I was dumbfounded. "What happened?" I asked.

"She was in a terrible car accident, Ray." Jonathan's demeanor was calm and soft, and his steady voice made you listen carefully. "When the paramedics came, they told me she was conscious and very calm. They said they were quite shocked by her behavior as they moved her into the ambulance. The paramedics both told me she looked happy and aware. Not losing her mind or hysterical. Not even in shock."

I squinted and listened more attentively.

"As the paramedics were rushing her to the hospital, they said at one point she sat up from the stretcher. She took the oxygen mask off her face and, in a lucid and gentle voice, said, 'I'm going to leave my body now. Hare Krishna, Hare Krishna, Krishna Krishna, Hare Hare.' And she left, Ray. The paramedics said they'd never seen anything like it."

"Oh my God. That's tragic . . . and wonderful . . . and horrible . . . and so wonderful." I didn't know what else to say, so I just shut up.

"In this world, Ray, there is danger at every step. We must always keep the holy name on our tongue. Then Krishna will take care of us."

*　　*　　*

In addition to the charm of Europe, the tour consisted of great shows, horrible shows, a riot in Belgium, and serendipitous meetings with spiritual people. I visited a few Krishna temples and even went to some Krishna restaurants. I reflected on what I wanted to do and where I wanted to live. After about two and a half months of touring, we headed back home.

While we were gone, my swan song record *Shelter* had started getting more and more attention in the music scene, and although we were not a band, we kept getting offers to play gigs. In my heart, I had left that scene behind. But it came after me. The more I read the *Gita*, the more

I understood that I had to face off with what I was in this life. I could not be something that I wasn't. So, I did something unprecedented in the sacred bhakti lineage—I started a band, a punk/hardcore band of celibate monks and Krishna devotees. We took the name of my solo record and called ourselves Shelter. It was loud, posthardcore, 1990s alternative music that the fans of Youth of Today were really into.

The more I studied these Vedic teachings the more I understood the true middle path. It was not renunciation of our gifts. It was using our gifts in a divine way. To renounce those would be a *dis*grace. A dis to God.

After connecting with other musical monks and swamis, I traveled across the United States from Potomac, Maryland, to Houston, Texas, then to San Diego, where Shelter officially became a band. We booked a tour around the States and landed in an ashram in an area of Philadelphia called Mount Airy.

The band was made up of me and some other brahmacharis who were also into music. Krishna Chaitanya, or K. C., was a cultured musician, a rock 'n' roll guy turned monk. Not punk at all. He listened to and loved Steely Dan, Pink Floyd, and Genesis, but he was a talented bass player and a great singer for backup vocals. He was humble and sincere and liked the idea of using his musical talents in service outside of kirtan, which he led excellently. I grabbed him in San Diego, where he lived in the ashram. He was well trained in studying sacred literature, and he inspired me to memorize chapters of the *Bhagavad Gita* in Sanskrit and English. K. C. could expertly play all the Indian instruments, including the mridanga, karatalas, and harmonium. So could Ekendra, our drummer, a multitalented musician and monk with a sweet, soft personality. He could also cook anything, anywhere. Because the monks in our tradition do not eat food cooked by non-Brahmins (as the consciousness of the cook enters the food), we brought a portable candy stove and a tank of propane wherever we went, and Ekendra would bust it out and make a feast for us within moments. We always traveled with moong dal, an array of Indian spices, and a five-gallon bucket of basmati rice. Ekendra was drawn to bhakti, but as a brahmachari never fulfilled his musical talents and was eager to join the band. Vic played guitar. He had toured in a band with Zack de la Rocha and was a great guitarist and a preacher of Vedic thought.

Ravindra Svarupa Prabhu, a wise married man in his fifties, ran the ashram. He had a PhD in religion from Temple University and a great sense of humor. He would teach us every morning, and it was like going to a university. His depth of both Eastern and Western philosophy gave us further depth in our own convictions and understandings. He also demonstrated how a family man like himself can be in this world but not of it.

He welcomed the band and appreciated our interesting way of sharing bhakti. He pretty much gave us carte blanche in the eight-thousand-square-foot mostly empty temple. Although A. C. Bhaktivedanta Swami had popularized the Krishna movement in the 1970s, by the time we got to the Philly ashram, it was in disrepair and most of the monks had left. Although it was run-down and had little funding to support it, the temple was an old hunting lodge on a charming, gorgeous piece of property. Mature chestnut and oak trees towered over the driveway. Old mansions lined the street. It was the last building before the neighborhood dramatically switched to a disinvested and neglected area. The temple was on the line between heaven and hell, and we had our fair share of break-ins and vandalism. Sometimes, the temple would run out of money for heat in the winter, making our already cold showers even colder, since we had to step out into a frozen building. The temple never charged us anything to stay there, and they kindly hosted us as we brought new life to the few overseeing the maintenance of the building and property.

Shelter flourished there. We created a practice studio in the basement of the temple, soundproofing the room as best as we could so as not to disturb anyone. We turned one of the larger rooms on the third floor into our office, where we started Equal Vision Records and manufactured and produced our own LPs and cassettes. Steve Reddy, who had been an original roadie for Youth of Today and then became a farmer, moved to Philadelphia to manage the band. There were about eight of us monks working at the record company. We released our records and any other bands that we could fit into our genre of spiritualized punk. This is how I had modeled Revelation Records, but now we were doing it as monks. We were not doing it for ourselves; we were doing it as an offering. Whether we sold a lot or a little, we felt the message was blessed. We didn't see other bands or genres as competitors. We weren't striving for a position, wealth, or fame. We were just trying to live the *Gita*—work and try our best. Follow dharma. Leave the results up to God. Be satisfied in our effort. We weren't basking in popularity or chasing it. We were here to honor what we received and give that message to the fans. Our agenda was no longer about us. It was no longer about being the center; it was about serving the center. All the stuff the yogis warn us about—kama (desire), krodha (anger), moha (illusion), lobha (greed)—had no room to manifest. We weren't using our popularity for taking. Any popularity, fame, or success we got was held in check by giving it back to the center—the most famous Lord Krishna. Fans would visit us in the temple. We'd welcome them as we had learned from our trips to India: Please sit. Take prasad. Let's read together.

* * *

On South Street in Philadelphia, there was a restaurant called Govinda's run by a charming man named Hari. Hari was a phenomenal cook, kirtan leader, and public speaker. He was African American and about fifteen years older than me, and he could give a dynamic class on the *Bhagavad Gita*. He invited us to come down and do a satsanga, or spiritual get-together, every Wednesday night at Govinda's. South Street was the punk/hip alternative street in Philly.

First, we'd start with nagar sankirtan, or public chanting in the streets. Dressed in our humble monk robes, tilak on our foreheads, Indian shawls, and slip-on black shoes, we would gather in front of the café at 6:30 p.m. Twenty to thirty fans from the music scene dressed in '90s hardcore attire—extremely baggy jeans and hooded sweatshirts for the boys and baggy stovepipe pants and crop tops revealing navel piercings for the girls—would show up. My band played the kirtan instruments beautifully. I led, playing *whompers*—large brass pie-tin-shaped hand cymbals, like hi-hats on a drum set, that sizzled and gave a low end to the kirtan when you tapped them together. They were the metronome. K. C. and Ekendra played mridangas in perfect unison. What I once did through the town of Vrindavan, I was doing now for a much different audience—the downtown Philadelphia alternative music scene. High school and post-high school fans chanted, danced, and sang along with us in two lines, creating a parade down crowded South Street. Sometimes, the girls wore saris and the boys dhotis. Everyone would dance and chant enthusiastically, up and down the street, blowing the minds of shop owners, shoppers, spiked-haired punks in leather jackets, and tourists.

It was a strange mix for sure. Some of us were dressed like orthodox monks, some looked ready for the mosh pit on the Warped Tour, and some were a hybrid of both cultures. All of us lost our material minds as we danced down the street like we were in a music video—singing sacred mantras, smiling, and joyfully aloof from public opinion. Steve stayed at the back, handing out invites to Part II. Part II was when we returned to Govinda's and piled everyone plus more into a room where I'd lead chanting on a harmonium and give a lecture on the *Bhagavad Gita* for forty minutes. We'd end with a big kirtan in the tiny room on the third floor that would literally make the early-nineteenth-century building shake. It was a fire marshal's nightmare—and a young soul searcher's dream.

Then Devati Deva Das, or 3-D as we called him, another young punk gone monk, showed up with his Wednesday night offering that he'd been lovingly preparing all day. Devati would spend all day in the kitchen preparing for this. His fried curd, or tofu, and peas in tomato sauce, basmati rice, papadams, and sweet blueberry-vanilla halva had everyone intoxicated. We'd eat on the floor on paper plates, forty people packed into the room that held twenty. It was *the* place to be on a Wednesday night. Our fans who showed up would tell their friends, and it became a thing—growing each week.

Living in the Philly temple was one of the joys of my life. What it lacked in a smooth, running organization, it made up for in great company, singing, cooking, eating, cleaning, adventure, festivals, and camaraderie. That was its great gift to me and many others. There were always spiritually committed visitors coming and going through the Equal Vision office, perhaps stopping by for lunch or sleeping at the ashram on weekends when their parents would allow them.

*   *   *

The band ended up touring the United States and Europe that first year. Like the Youth of Today tour before it, it wasn't easy for me. All our strict regulations of rising early, sitting quietly to meditate on beads, and eating were thrown off by late nights, dirty clubs, nine-hour drives, and living in a Mercedes Sprinter. That being said, we adjusted. Instead of going to bed and rising early, we had to stay up late to perform, so we'd continue staying up until the next day and do our meditation at 2 a.m. We'd sleep in, and our driver would drive. Ashrams around Europe in Germany, Sweden, Italy, Hungary, Poland, Norway, Holland, Switzerland, and Vienna would bring sacred prasad to our shows, offering us loaves of bread, Indian curries, spiced dal, and pastries. The ashram in Milan threw us a spaghetti party after one show we did there.

When we got the chance, we'd stay at ashrams and farms all around Europe, feeling welcome and loved. Sometimes they'd set up speaking engagements where fans could meet me and the band. I'd give classes from the *Bhagavad Gita* to the few hundred fans who'd show up before the show to hear me speak; then the devotees would offer them complimentary prasad. I gained deep peace and satisfaction in this spiritual mood of hearing knowledge, giving knowledge, giving prasad with love, and trusting that Krishna would decide how big, famous, or puny I would become.

After the tour, I knew I needed to reconnect with India on pilgrimage, so a few of us from the band took our earnings and did just that. Unfortunately our roadie and good friend Bhakta Tony, a hardcore fan from San Francisco who had moved into the ashram, confided in me that he had to leave. Tony was three or four years younger than me, and he said his mind was not peaceful and that giving up pot and sex cold turkey was too much for him. I tried to plead with him. "You know that stuff will not satisfy you." He agreed, but I could tell his mind was made up. We embraced, and he left the ashram.

Sometimes temptation got so great that people chose to leave an ashram or disappear in the middle of the night, feeling too ashamed to tell anyone. I loved Tony, and knew he struggled to control his senses. Of course he did. We were all young men fighting the current of the material world. The entire world struggles to control the senses. I was happy he tried.

My bandmates and I left for India the next day. It was 1991.

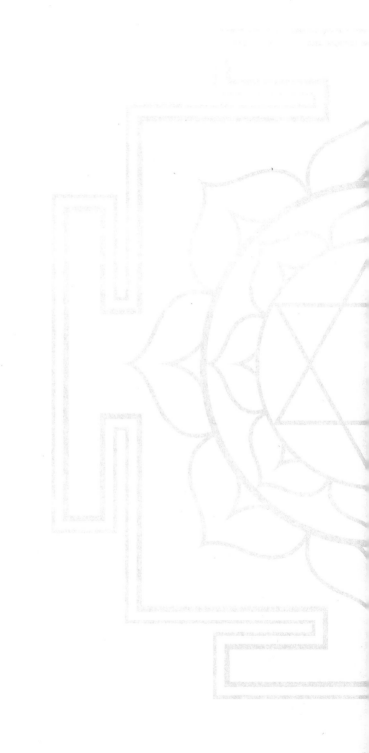

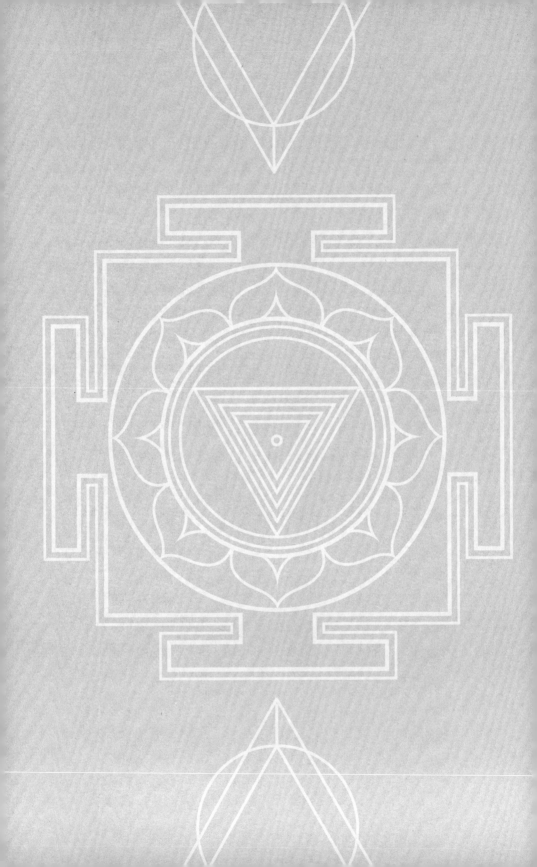

CHAPTER 9

TRANSCENDENTAL & TRAGIC ADVENTURES THROUGH INDIA

As soon as I arrived in Vrindavan, I met up with an old friend named Kaustubha, who I had known from hanging out in the New York City hardcore scene in the early 1980s. He used to be called Dave the Mod. Mods came from 1960s subculture, and they dressed cleanly and loved soul music. He had joined the ashram in NYC a year before me, in 1987, after having lost faith in the street music scene and had a higher calling when he met his guru during a class at the apartment of Harley Flanagan from Cro-Mags. He gave himself seriously to the ashram, traveling with a swami across the United States and becoming something of a missionary, dedicated to distributing the *Bhagavad Gita* wherever he went. Our paths would always magically cross without ever planning it, and sure enough, there we were—two punks from the Lower East Side in this holy land.

My first teacher, Swami-ji, who'd taken on a fatherly role when I first came to Vrindavan, had become a stable guide to go to if I had any questions regarding life choices, traveling in India, how to up my spiritual life, and of course the pitfalls on the path.

I asked him for diksha, or official connection to the spiritual tradition through initiation and vows. Although he didn't see himself as a guru, I insisted our relationship was already established in that way whether we liked it or not.

"You're all I have," I told him. "So can we make it official? Please?"

He consulted with an older guru he respected from Mathura, who insisted that taking on the role of guru was imperative so that the sacred holy mantras could be spread throughout the world.

On this trip in 1991, I took formal initiation and received the name Raghunath Das. I bowed down and received new mala beads that Swami-ji had chanted on. He explained that the name Raghunath is popular all over India because it's a name of Lord Rama. "But *you* are named after a young saint called Raghunath Das, who had everything of the material world one could dream of, but at a young age gave it all up to live in the jungles of Vrindavan and focus on God realization. He had no other desires in this world and was living in bliss. Follow in the footsteps of such great souls as Raghunath Das. Be convinced that the material world has nothing substantial to offer you. Continue to choose spiritual life over material life, and your life will be divine. Your name will be Raghunath *Das*, meaning servant of the great souls, like this Saint Raghunath."

Kaustubha's guru, Goswami Maharaj, also sat in on the initiation. He had been an instrumental person in my life, encouraging me when Shelter was just starting. He was also one of my teachers when I came to Vrindavan. Besides sacred literature, he also taught me how to cook, and for one month I became his personal servant and cook. He also initiated four people and gave Kaustubha the sacred thread, or the second initiation, which Vaishnavas receive after a certain amount of study and which gives one the privileges of secret and esoteric mantras to worship the deity on the altar in the temples. After the initiation, both of our formal teachers took us to the sacred Yamuna River to bathe, almost as a baptism into our new names and new spiritual identity.

The following day, we went to the sacred Radha Kunda and Shyama Kunda, villages at the tip of the sacred Govardhana Hill with two lakes, or bathing tanks as they call them in India. They were spring-fed ponds with sandstone steps on four sides descending toward the center like an inverted pyramid. They say that these holy bathing spots can grant one love of God as well as fulfill all desires. The entire village was peppered with ashrams. We went to visit different temples and ashrams and eventually sat down next to the sacred pond of Radha Kunda and took our bath, submerging ourselves in the love-laden waters. When we sat on the steps, we offered prayers for our friends, family, those who had gone astray, and those who needed direction. After all, they say Radha Kunda fulfills all desires and is considered a potent prayer vortex of sorts. Then I remembered Tony. I knew as soon as he left the temple that he would struggle. I knew maya well. Maya was like a baited trap, and the trap became more painful the more knowledge you had. In that holy spot I sincerely prayed for Tony to overcome all illusion, find new spiritual strength, get the hell out of San Francisco, and travel with us again on tour. By the time I got back to my room in Vrindavan, Bhakta Tony had magically appeared. I looked at him strangely, and then we both smiled and embraced.

"It's all true! This stuff really works!" I said in awe.

* * *

I loved my new name. It gave me a new sense of identity separate from my past. Tony and I were invited on a magical mystery tour of the beautiful northeastern Indian state of Manipur with the revered Bhaktisvarupa Damodara Swami. The rest of the band was traveling or studying on their own throughout India. Manipur was across the Bay of Bengal, adjoining Burma to the east and Bangladesh to the west. I had many adventures there, and the food was next level. I saw Vedic martial artist demos, which reminded me of silat, kali/eskrima, and other Indonesian and Filipino fighting styles, and the classical kirtan and dance was inspiring and impressive.

We headed back to Vrindavan on what should have been a seven-hour journey: one flight to Delhi then a four- to five-hour bus ride to Vrindavan, arriving in time for Gaura Purnima, the festival that celebrates the appearance of Sri Chaitanya Mahaprabhu, the Kirtan Avatar. Gaura Purnima is a wonderful day of song and feasting, but unreliable flights rerouted us to Kolkata, so I had to take a twenty-five-hour train ride to Delhi. I was livid at the incompetence of the transportation system and steeped with American arrogance and entitlement that only made me suffer more.

Everyone in India, especially the monks, had treated me with tolerance and compassion despite my being intolerant and entitled. Yet when I found myself sitting on this train journey opposite a belligerently drunk Indian man, who was mocking us, verbally abusive, and spitting when he spoke, every bone in my body wanted to hit him and tell him off. But I couldn't. I was sitting there dressed as a sadhu in my orange robes. Between when I'd left India four years ago and now, I had gotten more serious about my life as a renunciate. I was far from refined, but I was a work in progress. I had to remind myself that there was a new incarnation of myself that I was trying to step into.

How could I love this fool sitting across from me? First, I had to understand that he was possessed by tamo guna, or the mode of ignorance. He was intoxicated. Masking pain quickly and easily with cheap whiskey. My job as a practicing bhakta was not to give people their karma but rather to be tolerant, compassionate, and loving. I was a junior sadhu, a transcendentalist-in-training. I was *not* the administrator of karma to others. Let the universe chop people down or build them up. Let the universe take care of other people's karma. Not me.

Compassion. Tolerance. Love. That was my only job.

So I sat there and chanted and tolerated. Deep breathing. I started to think things through: *I'm sitting here, chanting. I'm learning Sanskrit verses from wisdom literature. Why? Why am I chanting anyway? It's a prayer for God to help me become tolerant, compassionate, and loving. So God, the universe, sweet baby Krishna—whatever you want to call Him—has sent someone specifically for me to work on my stuff. Why am I worried about this guy's stuff? What's my stuff? I'm not tolerant, compassionate, and loving. I'm short-tempered and cynical. Why should I get angry at this guy? I've been praying for him! I've been chanting for him to come. He's heaven sent! I'm singing loudly in kirtan for lessons to help me evolve. The universe has given me this crazed man for my benefit, to work on my stuff. How beautiful. How beautiful God is.*

This correction of my thought process was a beautiful challenge on that train ride. Whenever the train stopped, we had to be careful. It was Holi time in India, the day of throwing colored powders or colored water on anybody that walked by. Sometimes teenagers would come on the train and spray people with powder or giant water pistols. At one stop, two teenagers put a massive hose to the grated window of the train and pointed it at my head. I quickly slammed the window, and they adroitly aimed the hose toward the seat across from me, turned it on, and blew the drunken man off his seat with a high-powered stream of water. Miraculously, I was completely dry. Holi.

* * *

The train continued its seemingly endless journey. I walked past people and families sitting on the floor on my way to the train toilets. The one on the left had a sign that read "Western style," indicating you'd be sitting on a commode. I chose the Indian style. Better ergonomics when working with sandals and robes. It was a small prison cell of sorts. The toilet plumbing was quite simple. It was an open hole onto the railroad tracks. Why not?

Every other animal defecates outside. We've created elaborate chemical systems using and wasting potable water to flush waste into holding tanks. "Flushing" it away doesn't make it go away. It goes somewhere. Waste-treatment plants use chemicals, which make their way back into the water table. In the name of fixing problems, we create new ones.

India hadn't figured this one out yet, either. Half of the population didn't have access to waste-management systems, but I didn't believe the Western fix was the way to go—it just flushed a bigger mess under the rug.

I reached into my shoulder bag to grab my toilet paper, and after doing my business, I washed my hands using my Dr. Bronner's soap. Then I headed back to my berth. There had been a change of passengers in my absence. Now a poor, simple, yet clean sadhu sat in my seat. He had matted hair and a thick Vaishnav tilak on his forehead. I sat next to him. His skin was smooth, and he wore one strand of thick tulasi beads around his neck. His eyes were sweet from a lifetime of a disciplined mind.

"Hello, my son," he said in perfect English. He was carrying very little. He had a small shoulder bag and a beautiful, smooth walking stick.

"Jai Sri Krishna," I said. It was my common salutation. All glory to Lord Krishna. Any sect of Hinduism could appreciate that statement.

"You are a Krishna bhakta?"

I nodded. "I'm trying to be."

"Yes," he chuckled. "We are all trying. But in that trying Lord Krishna sees your bhakti and will come to you. Bhagavan Krishna does not care much about your intelligence. You may be very intelligent, but that is not enough to catch Krishna. And sweet Krishna does not care if you are a wealthy man. That does not catch Him either. By material means this young boy is very difficult to catch." He looked around and got close to me as if telling me a secret, "Yashoda Maiya . . . do you know?"

I nodded, as he was about to tell me a Krishna story about Krishna's mother, Yashoda.

"Krishna's mata was also very fond of him, you could imagine, but Krishna was angry at her for putting Him down when she was cooking milk on the stove. Young Krishna got very mad and crawled into the other room, where mother Yashoda kept the clay pots of butter and curd," he said, using the British way of saying yogurt. "Little Krishna picked up a stone and threw it at the pot, which was hanging from the rafters of the house."

I nodded, playing dumb, although I knew the story. I just wanted him to tell it to me, as I found him incredibly charming. His eyes were glowing, and his eyebrows lifted. "Please continue," I said.

"Lord Krishna broke that pot of butter, and his mother got very angry. 'Where is this naughty boy?' she asked angrily and searched hither and thither for him. She found him, his face covered with butter, sitting in a pool of butter and feeding it to the monkeys. 'Just see my naughty son. Now I will teach you a lesson!' she said furiously. She went to fetch some rope from the kitchen to tie Krishna to a big spice mortar. When she tried to tie up the boy, she discovered her rope was two fingers too short. Frustrated, she went to get more rope to teach her son a lesson, and after tying the two ropes together, she found that this rope was still two fingers too short! *How could this be?* she thought. She went and got multiple ropes and tied them together, and when she went to tie young Krishna, she still found this mysterious phenomenon—the rope was still two fingers too short! She was shocked! She sat down in despair. At this time, Krishna, sensing his mother's love through her chastisement, allowed her to tie him up. Those two fingers represented endeavor and grace. This is how we catch God. We try to approach with love. That's our endeavor. And then God's grace allows.

"Young Krishna is only caught by love. When you do catch him, he never lets you go, either. Krishna is like that. You think you are mad after Krishna? No, no! He is *mad* after you! He falls deeply in love and in debt to his bhakta."

This man's childlike charm lit up my heart. This is the real wealth I came to find in India. This destitute man was joyful with nothing. Voluntarily renouncing the world, he had a gorgeous simplicity and joy. Having nothing but God, he seemed to have everything.

* * *

When Tony and I finally got to Delhi, we moved quickly to try to get to the bus station. The station was an unbelievable sight for my American eyes. People were sleeping everywhere! I wasn't sure if they were beggars, sadhus, travelers, or homeless. But the incredibly cheap fare of less than $1 made us choose this instead of a $40 taxi ride. We were monks. This is how we should travel.

In the back of my mind I knew I was getting some royalties from my band and could afford a taxi, but I felt it was more appropriate for a sadhu in training to tolerate and travel inexpensively and give my earnings in charity. Communication was tricky, as the ticket man for the bus didn't speak English. By that time it was 1 a.m., and I was exhausted. I went to the booth and tried with my best Hinglish to find out when the next bus was leaving for Mathura. Tony was sleeping on our little bags on the ground. From what I understood, the man told me that at 3 a.m. the bus would leave from gate 32 and the bus was there waiting now. I woke up Tony. We bought some hot peanuts, which we loved, from the peanut wallah and some dehydrated mango squares, another great roadside food. We grabbed our stuff and walked over to the gate.

The place was filthy, and after traveling on that train for twenty-five hours, so were we. We thought that since the bus was parked there, maybe they'd let us get on and sleep in it. These buses fill up, so we thought it best to tie our luggage to the roof and get on early. I confirmed with the driver, "Mathura–Agra bus 3 a.m.? Teen baji?" I asked, looking for a reasonable confirmation.

He nodded.

There was a makeshift ladder on the side of the bus, and we climbed up. We carefully tied our backpacks down to the roof, using some extra shoelaces we had. Sometimes people just travel on the roof of buses when they are overcrowded. I've never done that. Tony and I sat on that roof eating peanuts, looking at the night sky.

"Ever think of what's going on up there? How arrogant we are to think that life merely exists here on this planet," I said.

"What do the Vedas say about life on other planets?" he asked.

"Living beings are everywhere in different bodies. The bodies may not look like our bodies, but they exist throughout the universe. Some planets they say are earthly, with both good and bad situations. Some are heavenly planets for the pious, and they're filled with great types of sense pleasure, long lives, and no disease. Some are painful places, like what the Christians call hell. But *all* the planets are temporary homes, meaning we go there, spend some time, learn some lessons if we're lucky, and hopefully evolve. Of course, sometimes we don't evolve—we devolve. This is all the material universe," I said, pointing to the sky. "Both Hindus and Buddhists call our situation samsara. Spinning around, making choices. Hopefully, we meet some people that help us make good choices. Often, we meet people that influence us to make bad choices. And if we're very fortunate, we meet mahatmas, or great souls who help us make transcendental choices to escape the cycle.

"Higher, lower, and middle planets. *Om bhur bhuvah sva*, the *Gayatri Mantra* says. We're just here to learn lessons. Spiritual life is not about complaining about our situation, but understanding how we are here to grow from everything in our path."

Tony was a few years my junior, and he lay back on the roof of the bus and listened as I played the role of a junior guru for a moment. The bus roof was a great vantage point to see the terminal, the sky, and the city. It was a crappy tin can of a vehicle, made cheaply. Nothing like a Greyhound bus from the States. This bus looked as if there were no rules for making buses here. No standards. No plans or blueprints. As if welded by a bunch of teenagers in a metal shop. I was once on a bus with a driver who wrapped himself in chadars, or shawls, and wore a winter hat because there was no windshield. There was something shocking, yet beautiful, about the lawlessness—it appealed to my punk-rock sensibility.

We lay on that roof, looking up at the sky, thinking about life on other planets, and popping peanuts in our mouths, for about twenty minutes. Then we heard the bus start—a couple of hours before we expected it to leave. People rushed to get on.

Weird! I thought. *The driver just told me it was leaving at 3 a.m.*

I tilted my head over the side of the bus and banged on the window as he was starting to pull out. "Wait!" I screamed. "Bus to Agra and Mathura teen baji?"

"Yes, but leaving now instead," he replied.

"Only in India can you just reschedule the bus without letting anyone know," I mumbled.

"With people on the roof!" Tony said.

We jumped down from the bus before it could take off. It was packed. We found two seats next to each other in the middle toward the back. No padding. No headrest. No comfort. Tolerance. I breathed deep. This would be a four-hour bus ride on a one-lane potholed road. Tony put his forehead to rest on the metal rim of the seat in front of him. Out of sheer exhaustion, he fell asleep immediately.

Cars sped at us, the drivers with one hand on the horn, blaring constantly, and one hand on the wheel. This made the ride a cacophony of discordant honks and air horns. The speeding vehicles, including ours, drove right at each other as though we were all playing chicken. At the last moment, both vehicles would pull to their respective sides of the road, barely missing a head-on collision. *Better to not even look*, I thought. The usual goatherds—even at 2 a.m.—were also on the road, which caused the bus to make abrupt stops and swerves. An occasional camel cart broke our pace as well.

After a thirty-plus-hour journey, I was exhausted, too, and fell asleep. After about two hours, we were awakened when the bus shrieked to a firm stop. There was confusion, yelling, crying, and screaming. Flares and temporary lights shone outside. We immediately became alert, as though somebody had poured a bucket of cold water on our heads. A large truck carrying chickens had hit an ox cart and a passenger bus slightly smaller than ours. The ox was lying on his back, practically upside down and definitely dead. I could see its ghastly form through the bus windshield, a scene lit by our headlights and the flashlights and lanterns of local villagers. The chicken truck was on its side, and chickens were flying and squawking everywhere. Then I realized it was grimmer than that. People were trapped beneath the passenger bus, and the villagers were rocking the bus to free the victims.

"What the hell is going on?" Tony shouted.

Tony and I just looked at each other. We couldn't digest what was going on. The frantic energy was trumped only by the village people, who started bringing bodies, some critically injured and some dead, onto our bus. The severely injured lay unconscious in the aisle. The villagers had turned our bus into a makeshift ambulance/hearse. Bodies writhing in pain, or still and corpselike, lined the entire aisle.

Tony and I were both pale. We didn't know what to do. We didn't even know where we were. The sounds of moaning and screaming surrounded us, like a haunted house. A bawling lady came on the bus with a blood-soaked towel over her face, and someone helped her sit down in the front seat—the passengers pushed in tighter to accommodate her. From what I understood, we were about to head to some hospital, which might add several hours to our trip. Between the howling, the screaming, the dead ox, the chickens, the blood, and not being able to understand the language,

Tony and I started freaking out. But we were trapped. There was no room to get out of the vehicle. The aisles were packed with bodies. Our bags were on the roof. Vrindavan was at least two hours away.

"What the hell are we going to do?" Tony looked at me desperately.

I didn't know. So, we shimmied our bodies out a postage stamp of a window. There were no emergency exit windows, like the ones on US buses. I grabbed onto the roof rail and got myself up to the top of the bus to untie our stuff. Tony followed. Then the engine started.

"Untie quicker!" Tony said.

"I tied it with this shoelace, and it's in a granny knot! I cannot undo it!"

Tony jumped with his bag off the side and tried to tell the driver to wait, pointing to me on the roof. I finally snapped the string by force. I banged on the windshield to stop the driver, then jumped off, using the side-view mirror as a giant step. The bus zipped off for its emergency drive to the local hospital.

Tony and I sat down on a bench near a closed roadside stand. Our heads were spinning. There was still commotion. Chickens. The dead ox. Blood. Glass. People with minor injuries. The locals were still rocking the bus, trying to get it back upright on four wheels. They did it skillfully, as if they had done it before. They had already done the same for the chicken truck. I checked my watch—4 a.m.

I looked at a rickshaw driver. "Where is Vrindavan? How far?" I asked in my broken Hindi.

"One hour," he replied.

The scene was calming down. A lady started heating up a big wok of chai for all the villagers that were helping. The smell of ginger and buffalo milk grounded me. I felt like I was having an out-of-body experience. We were exhausted but only an hour away from Vrindavan.

"We could have been one of those dead bodies," Tony said.

"It might have been worse to be one of the injured bodies," I said. "I've never heard cries of agony like that before. God knows the hospitals around here must be totally budget." I remembered the verse I was studying on the train and shared it with Tony:

> For those who have accepted the boat of the lotus
> feet of the Lord, who is the shelter of the cosmic
> manifestation, the ocean of the material world is like
> the water contained in a calf's hoof-print. Their goal
> is param padam, Vaikuntha, the place where there
> are no material miseries, not this world where there
> is danger at every step.

"Yes," Tony said, "there's danger at every step in the material world. Death comes in a moment! None of those people on the bus thought, *Today I will die.* None thought, *Today I will be maimed!*"

Tony was in a state of shock. I ordered two cups of chai, and we sat and drank them. Both of us were thinking of our own temporality. We thought of our frail existence. There was something about India that didn't cover up the realities of life. The beauty was real. So was the death, disease, and pain. The most materialistic and the most spiritual. The most refined and the most grotesque. Nothing was glossed over. It was all available to witness. To inhale. To drink in.

I thought about my father's death. About the poor souls that died in the bus crash. The air was still biting from the morning cold, and it was foggy. We sat on strangely comfortable wooden benches, sipping chai from clay cups. I started to talk to Tony about spiritual truths.

"We are living in this world with a time bomb strapped to us," I said. "A time bomb that is set to go off, but we don't know when. Most people hide the time bomb under their shirt and ignore it. They fill their lives with diversions. Diverting their mind from the ticking of the bomb of death. They divert it with material goals, romance, adventure, desires for fame, popularity, or economic development. Anything to forget that tick, tick, ticking. That inevitable death. Anything except looking at that bomb—our brittleness. We fill our minds with anything to ignore the fact that there's something ticking underneath our shirt. Some people are neurotic about the time bomb. Some are in denial. True escapism."

"And people say spiritualists are escapists who have their heads buried in the sand."

"Yes, it's the total opposite. If we can meditate and keep our fallibility and our vulnerability at the forefront of our mind, then there's hope that we can turn inward toward spirit. As spiritual seekers we have to be somewhere in between. We need to recognize death is real and is coming at any moment. Like the verse says, 'There's danger at every step.' We need to focus on our real self and move forward on our path. Once we can pop the romantic bubble of maya of the material world, we can develop sobriety from the illusion of life."

It felt good to say this. It encapsulated and gave some closure to the grisly scenes we had just witnessed.

"I like that, Prabhu! Tony said. "Spiritual sobriety!"

We cheers'd our clay cups and drank some more chai. I asked a motor rickshaw wallah how much it would be to take us to Vrindavan. Without haggling I accepted the 400-rupee price and we jumped in, still holding our warm drinks. I wrapped my wool chadar around my shoulders and ankles and sat in sukhasana pose to protect me from the biting morning cold. The rickshaw started shooting out bellows of black diesel exhaust.

"Vrindavan quickly!" I said in Hindi with a smile. The driver gave a head bobble to acknowledge me, and we headed out on that deserted road, wide awake and ready to reenter our spiritual home.

* * *

Holi, also called the Festival of Colors, takes place for nine days each spring in Vrindavan. The color and water throwing is supposed to be a sweet gesture of loving teasing of one another, as Radha and Krishna would some-times squirt each other with syringes—old-school water pistols filled with colored water. People give Holi different meanings. Some say it represents the colors of spring. Some say it's considered a day of triumph of good over evil, as Holika, the evil sister of the demon king Hiranyakashipu, was killed in a fire on that day. People build a ceremonial fire to pray that their personal internal evil will be destroyed.

In modern times, at least in northern India where I was, it was one month of utter chaos—getting attacked with colored water, water guns, and exterminator sprayers filled with dye and water. Kids threw buckets of colored water at any moment. Everyone was fair game—old, young, men, women, tourists, locals. The color extravaganza was usually a playful mood where there was no room for ego or bravado. If you're on the street, anywhere, you're getting covered in dye whether you like it or not.

I had too much of an ego, so I stayed on the temple grounds where they didn't allow the color throwing. The problem, though, was that Tony woke up ill one morning. He had stomach cramps and a fever. He asked me to pick up some medicine for him down the road at the market. He looked pathetic and exhausted. Of course, I would do it. A friend in need is a friend indeed. I walked out of the front gate of the ashram. As soon as I stepped out of the gate, a young girl no older than ten came up to me with a squirt gun and shot me in the cheek. Blue water dripped down my ear and onto my saffron kurta, leaving stains on my face and shirt. I quickly jumped on a rickshaw and gave the driver the address without even bargaining for the price.

"Quickly, quickly move!" I yelled in Hindi. Too late—a teenager took a soaked red cloth and smacked it across my head. I didn't like my personal space invaded. The New Yorker in me got pissed off, and I was ready to kick some ass. But I was a monk. I couldn't do that. Another kid, with green dye, hit me with a sponge on the top of my head. I felt humiliated as he and a bunch of friends laughed. I watched in the distance as a bus was flagged down. A teenager got on with a bucket of blue water and threw it on the passengers. "Holi!" he shouted, laughing. No one cared. In fact, all the older pilgrims on the bus acted like they had been blessed by the pope or something.

This is out of control! I thought. I tried to imagine a Greyhound bus getting stopped on the streets of New York City with some kid throwing a bucket of blue water on the passengers. It would never fly.

My rickshaw took off quickly, but three teenagers got in some last squirts of red water on my robe, face, and arm. Fortunately, we sped up and were going fast enough not to be a target. We dodged meandering cows, a herd of goats, horse-drawn tongas, and other rickshaws. My driver was fast, and probably could have made it to the Olympics, considering the strength of his thighs! I was also soaking wet from the colored water. My robe hung awkwardly, as if it wanted to disrobe itself from my body. We rode on, and the hot wind from the fast-moving rickshaw cooled me off in the noon heat.

Besides a few run-ins with stray pigs, a bull, and some pedestrians, we made it smoothly to the market, which is called Loi Bazaar. It was filled with tiny shops selling unique items: cloth, brass, oil lamps, deities, silver, copper, incense, wooden beads, you name it. Of course, there were fruit vendors, fried snack vendors, and men stirring big woks and making sweetmeats, delicious Indian milk sweets. Burfi, chum-chums, gulab jamun, kala jamun, laddu, jalebi, the list goes on and on. I tried them all.

The shops were no bigger than a small room, with thin mattresses of white cloth on the floor. You had to take off your shoes and step up into the open shops, which were raised about three feet from the ground. The shopkeepers, working with their children, called in customers by saying, "Jai Radhey! Hari Bol! Prabhu! Please come!" Usually they slapped the mat and said, "Sit down!" Oftentimes, they brought you a drink, like a lassi or nimbu pani (fresh lemonade) served in clay cups—real customer service that made you want to hang out and spend money.

I just needed some simple constipation medicine, some chyavanprash (an Ayurvedic herbal jam), and some aspirin. The shopkeeper knew me. "Nothing else, Mr. Raghunath?" he said, encouraging a bigger purchase. "Chandrika soap, Vicco toothpaste, tongue scraper, perhaps?" He knew I was a sucker for Ayurvedic products.

"No, I'm fine, it's not for me. My friend is not well," I replied.

"Panch minute, Prabhu-ji. I am getting some chyavanprash from my warehouse. Sit down. You want lassi?" Without waiting for a reply, he sent his seven-year-old son to fetch me a delicious frothy yogurt shake.

I sat on a bench. When he said to wait five minutes, I knew I was going to be there for a while. Indian time ran much differently than American time. I sat comfortably, safe from the Holi color war going on outside, and reached for my journal.

Across the street were a bunch of monkeys hanging out on top of the shops. I loved watching them. Scheming. Like a street gang. The more I watched them, the more I started peering into the minds of the monkeys. They were hiding above the fruit vendor, waiting for innocent people to purchase fruit, and then they would attack, steal the fruit, and swiftly run back up a lamppost to the roof. This happened repeatedly, just a few feet over the head of the shopkeeper but back far enough that he couldn't get them. One monkey jumped onto a man's back and took his wallet. The monkey, jumping *just* out of reach, feigned giving the wallet back. Then he opened the wallet, took out the rupees, and tore them in half. If I didn't see this with my own eyes, I wouldn't have believed it.

"These Vrindavan monkeys are not ordinary," the shopkeeper said, seeing me amused. "They were great sages that did some naughty behavior here and had to take one more birth before being liberated. This is why we tolerate their behavior. They are not ordinary souls. It is like Maharaja Bharata."

He was referring to the story of a great king, Bharata, who was very spiritually evolved but not yet perfected. The king left for the forest on the bank of a holy river to prepare for death, regularly doing his rituals, mediations, and puja. One day he saw a pregnant deer drinking from the river while he was sitting peacefully. Suddenly the deer, hearing the frightening roar of a lion, gave birth to a fawn, which got swept down the river. King Bharata, breaking his meditation, instinctually ran after the helpless creature and rescued it. (The mother deer, unfortunately, was killed by the lion.) He took the fawn back to his humble ashram and let it rest, and the baby got attached to the king as a surrogate mother. The king also got attached to the young deer. He eventually gave up his meditation to spend more time with the deer. Although we may forget death, death does not forget us, and King Bharata died in meditation not on Lord Vishnu but on the fawn. Because of this, he was reincarnated as a deer.

I thought about all the children in this town growing up chanting and singing in kirtan. All the pilgrims. All the dogs, pigs, cows, and even trees. They were all growing up with an entire town speaking and singing about Krishna all day. The animals were being fed leftovers of sacred prasad. Who were they previously that they ended up on this hallowed ground? *Yes,* I thought, *these may not be ordinary monkeys.*

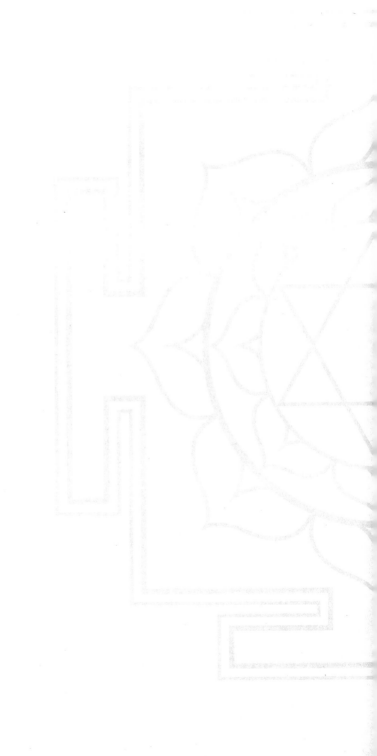

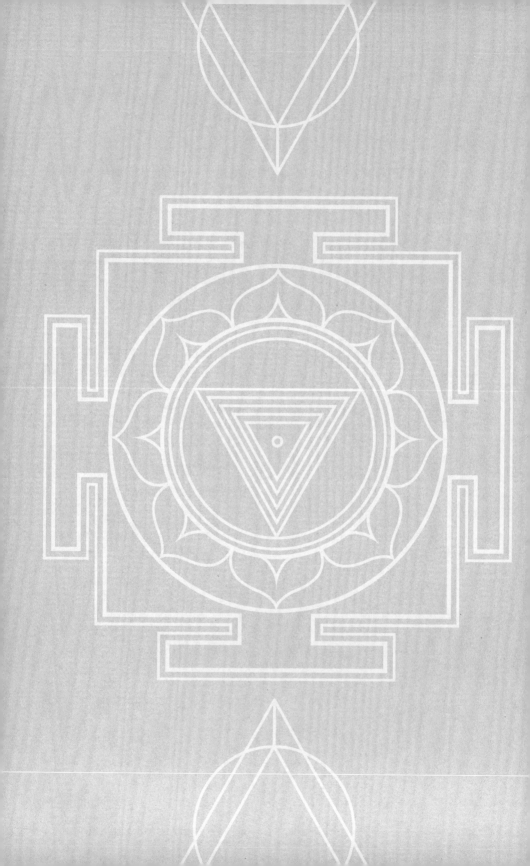

CHAPTER 10

BLENDING MONKHOOD & MUSIC

When I returned to the United States, I heard that Porcell, without my direct influence, had decided to become a monk. It was hard to believe because he never seemed to have spiritual inclinations. He was already straight edge, health conscious, worked in health food stores, and had a good heart, and I was sure he was exhausted with the trappings of the music world, just as I had been.

He gave up Judge, the influential international band he formed after I left for India the first time. He renounced a Gibson Les Paul guitar for the orange robes of a renunciate and moved to the same rural Pennsylvania farm ashram where Steve lived. When I returned to Philly and heard this news, I drove out to the farm and begged him to give up farm life and pick up the guitar again, this time using it for service instead of self. After consulting with seniors, he gave in and joined Shelter. This new lineup toured the world, keeping the Philly ashram as our base and frequenting India every year for a spiritual refueling.

It became too hard to concentrate and focus to write a new record at the temple. I was frustrated, distracted, and overwhelmed. I needed a place where I could just sit and write music and lyrics for hours without fans or devotees walking in. Steve Reddy recommended that I disappear somewhere to write music. But where? I was a monk. I wanted accountability and good company. Then I received a perfect invite from Bhakta Henry.

I met Henry in 1988, when I was twenty-two, on my first trip to India. His white Mercedes and driver pulled into Vrindavan. He was only about ten years older than me, but he came from an old-money family in the United States. He was a genuine searcher and proclaimed that he was "on many paths, just not sure which one yet." We bonded. We were both anomalies—weirdos of sorts walking around holy lands with holy people. We shared rickshaws, prasad, personal struggles, and spiritual desires.

Now, four years later, Henry loved that I was in a punk band for Krishna. He grew up in Washington, D.C., a prodigal son, hanging with his older brother and partying with the likes of Led Zeppelin, the Rolling Stones, and Andy Warhol. He even worked in a pet store with Henry Rollins. But his inner calling was louder, and the party scene unfulfilling. In 1982, he got hooked on going to India. It was his sixth time there when I met him.

Now he called to invite me to visit him in Washington, D.C. because he heard I may need space and time to practice, demo, and write new music. It was a Krishna miracle, and just in the nick of time.

I had been to his house—an old, massive home packed with European antiques in the exclusive Embassy Row district of Washington, D.C.—a few years earlier. Large oil paintings of his family members going back centuries, statues, busts, delicate furniture, chandeliers. It was like moving through a museum that was both charming and creepy. He warmly invited the entire band to come down for a month or two, whatever it took to finish our new record.

When our van pulled up into the neighborhood, we were surprised by the house. In the few years since I had visited Henry, he had painted it a pretty light saffron, the same shade as our monk robes—not what you'd expect on a house in the upscale neighborhood. It popped. Henry opened the door and welcomed us, and when I walked in, I was even more surprised. None of his family heirlooms were there. No more massive oil paintings or statues. Most of the furniture was gone. The entire place was redone—it was bright, uplifting, and inspiring and felt like a celestial ashram. Gorgeous original Rajasthani paintings and colorful tapestries adorned the walls. Sitting cushions and bolsters were on the floor, and bookshelves of sacred literature lined the walls. I could tell Henry was going through a spiritual transformation similar to mine.

"What happened to your home?" I asked. "I mean, I always liked it but it . . . it's beautiful now. I feel like I'm in the spiritual world."

"You become like who you associate with, Raghu," said Henry. "I've had two incredible guests staying with me for almost a year now, and I can honestly say they've deeply changed me in a wonderful way. You're going to love them, and they're going to love you. I've prepared a studio on the bottom floor for you to practice in. It's totally soundproofed and ready for you. I even have some guys that can help you load in your gear and help you get set up."

Two men appeared out of nowhere, ready for some heavy lifting.

The rest of the band was awestruck, just looking around the massive house and zeroing in on the artwork. Henry broke into art curator mode. "They're all original works by B. G. Sharma from Udaipur, India. He's a Rajasthani master. Just look at the details." The details were incredible. It was fine, intricately crafted artwork that used minerals, shells, plants, and even precious stones as vibrant paint.

"The old version of your house looked like a European museum, but this remodel looks like a palace temple!"

"Thank you," he said politely. "My houseguests have made you all lunch."

"Who are your houseguests?" Now I was curious.

Out walked two stunning ladies, probably in their late forties. I recognized Yamuna Devi, a world-famous personal chef, immediately. She was A. C. Bhaktivedanta Swami's personal chef, traveling with him all over India and the world. The swami personally taught her to cook, and she went on to write an award-winning, internationally best-selling cookbook titled *Lord Krishna's Cuisine*. She also recorded a hit record with George Harrison and, in fact, was one of the people that introduced George and John Lennon to bhakti in the 1970s.

The other woman, her friend Dina Tarine, I did not know. She was not as known as Yamuna but just as spiritually stellar. We were bhakti starstruck.

"We're honored to have the boys from Shelter here. My name is Yamuna Devi, and this is Dina. I'm working on my new cookbook every day, and I humbly ask you to try all of my recipes and let me know if they are good enough to put in the new book. Would that be okay?"

Needless to say, we immediately fell in love with these women. Especially after Yamuna brought us into the kitchen and we tried some food, including a chiffon cake.

Every morning we'd gather around Yamuna as she did her predawn worship of her deities. She, with an angelic voice, led us in kirtan. Then she'd open the *Bhagavad Gita* and teach a class like a pandit, including personal stories of her traveling with her guru, many of which we hadn't heard before. This happened every day. Singing. *Gita*. Eating her offerings. Taste-testing for her new book. Listening to her stories of the early days of bhakti in the United States and India in the 1970s, traveling with the Beatles.

On our third day, Yamuna made a wonderful refined Indian feast using the most delicate spicing. She told us how A. C. Bhaktivedanta Swami was an incredible connoisseur and had the palate to taste even the finest details of her cooking.

"Yamuna-ji," I complained, "I feel so uncultured and so American!"

"Why?"

"I just don't have a cultured palate. Your food is so refined, and all I want to do is pour ketchup and mustard on everything."

She laughed and gracefully took the chapatis off the cast-iron grill and deftly flipped them onto the open flame of the gas burner, where they puffed into perfect balls. Then she removed them from the heat and threw them on a small, covered plate so they'd stay warm. She brushed them with ghee, then used her tongs and tossed them onto our plates. It was quite an impressive display.

"Yamuna, this is prasad," said Dina. "You can't throw it around the kitchen!"

Yamuna smiled coyly, giving us a sweet head bobble. "She's right!" she said.

The next day during the meal, Yamuna pulled out a small pot of smooth tomato chutney. "This is for you, Raghunath. I've made it especially for you. For your uncultured palate. It's the ketchup you want to smother your food in." This was one of the sweetest gestures.

One day I went to her and told her that I didn't know if I would ever fit in a spiritual institution. "I'm too much of my own person."

She smiled and said, "Me too. But that's okay. We just need to take whatever we do and make it an offering with love. There's no box we need to fit in, Raghunath."

* * *

Henry had a bunch of video recording equipment and an editing system set up in his downstairs studio. I convinced him to follow us on a tour that we were about to embark on around the States, film us, and make a tour video. Henry, always up for the adventure, opted in almost immediately and followed our van in his Grand Cherokee.

Our first show was in Buffalo, New York, in a massive warehouse that turned out to be in a bad neighborhood. There were about four other bands there, and we were headlining the show. Hundreds of fans showed up, and we set up our van outside the warehouse where the kids were lined up, paying to get in. We sat on the ground singing sacred kirtan, while fans walked by us, mystified. A crowd gathered and watched us. Ekendra had cooked a massive pot of kitchari and offered some with love to our traveling altar. He distributed it in paper bowls the same way temples in India handed out sacred prasad to pilgrims. We also set up a massive merchandise table where we had shirts just like any other punk/hardcore band, but also pictures of Lord Vishnu with the words "SHELTER: self-realization not sense gratification" written on the back. This was our biggest seller. It was an incredible night. Not just because of sales but because of new relationships, the performance, the reception of the crowd. Everything was beautiful, nearly perfect.

Then, it all fell apart.

After the show, our roadies and most of the band members drove the van into the warehouse to load out our gear and the PA system. Henry was meandering around filming, and I was out in the alley where we'd had kirtan earlier, getting interviewed for a local magazine. Most of the teenage or twentysomething fans were heading home for the night.

During my interview, in my periphery, I saw a car pull up and six massive men get out. They didn't look like they were from our scene—they looked like criminals, up to no good. They immediately grabbed one of the concert goers, a young kid, and beat him ruthlessly. Fights break out at shows occasionally, but it's usually not from outsiders. I was getting interviewed, so I didn't flinch that much—until they stopped beating the kid and moved to another similarly small person. By the time they moved on to the third victim, people started scattering. After all, these guys were twice everyone's size and looked extremely dangerous. We were in a bad part of town, and it was 2:30 a.m. My interviewer left, and I ran inside to get the band and warn them that trouble was going down right outside the club. "You guys, we gotta get out of here."

The band looked at me and shrugged their shoulders. All our van doors were open, our gear was only half loaded, and the merchandise still wasn't broken down. "We can't leave now," said Tony.

Just then, I watched the thugs' car drive right up to the warehouse—perpendicularly in front of our van, barricading us inside. It was eerie. There were only about twenty of us left in the warehouse. The six guys got out of the car. The biggest, a hulk of a man, put his hand in his back pocket and pulled out a gun. He spoke in a serious, firm voice that instantly changed the atmosphere.

"I've got a gun. And I'm gonna kill everyone tonight!" It was like hearing the death knell. Our faces dropped, and a pit formed in my stomach. The goons went around the warehouse and continued beating random people. The band and roadies circled me, petrified and confused, and looked to me for a solution.

Why didn't we run, fight back, or scream? It was all too sudden, too fast, and the guys were too big and armed. I had only one answer, and I'm not sure where it came from. "We're going to die tonight," I said. "So, we're going to chant."

I went into the van and pulled out the drum we use for kirtan. The band obediently circled up with me. We started chanting prayers to Narasimha, the ferocious man-lion avatar of Vishnu famous for protecting his devotees.

The entire thing was surreal. Psychopaths were beating people in an empty warehouse at 2:30 a.m. in Buffalo, and we were standing in a circle singing Vedic mantras. If I wasn't there, I wouldn't have believed it. But my number came up next, and the gang came up to us. Immediately, and understandably, the band fled. K. C. hid under the van, Ekendra jumped in the van, screaming mantras, Henry hopped into the passenger seat ghost-faced, eyes wide open, perhaps not realizing what he'd signed up for. Everyone took off, and I ended up standing there holding an Indian drum, surrounded by six lunatics. Towering above me, the leader grabbed his gun from his back pocket, and said, "So, you want some?!"

I had no idea what was happening. I was still standing there, impotently, wearing a big drum around my shoulders. I looked the guy in the eyes, drew my hands to namaste, and said, "I am a devotee of Lord Krishna, and I have no idea why you guys are so angry."

That's when they began pummeling me. Fist after fist landed on my head, neck, and jaw. I had never felt helpless like this before. It was fist after fist after fist after fist. I can honestly say that then something mystical happened. It is written repeatedly in the lore of India that great souls ready to depart from their body drew their attention inward and either meditated on the form of Lord Vishnu or chanted. I had read about the auspicious passing of great souls as they left their mortal frame in a sober consciousness, free from fear and lamentation. It seemed almost romantic. In this moment of utter helplessness, I found myself chanting out loud, too. Every time I got slugged in the face, I called out a divine mantra. A name of the Absolute. "Krishna! Govinda! Rama! Madhava!" I screamed a name every time I was punched. I felt like one of those holy men in meditation. Amid the mayhem, I thought: *I'm getting beaten ruthlessly, but I'm chanting the holy name! This is incredible!*

At that moment, three women with baseball bats ran toward me. With false hope, I thought they were coming to save me. They must have been the girlfriends of the men that were beating me. The women hit me repeatedly with the bats. Three times in the head, once on the shoulder, once on the arm, and once on my thigh. Blood poured from my skull, covering my face, shoulders, shirt, and the drum I was still wearing. Magically, every time I was struck, every time that bat came down on my body, mantras poured out of my mouth. My inner voice spoke loudly in my head. I was being mystically coached: "You could have your skull split open, yet every time you get hit, you're chanting the holy name! You're not pure yet, these are potentially your last moments on this planet, and you're chanting fearlessly in full God consciousness! This is the perfection of your life!"

Somehow, instead of being scared, I was inspired. I couldn't explain it, and I knew I was not a very evolved soul, but I felt I was given a gift: a glimpse of what it was like to be one of those mahants, or great personalities that leave their body with an evolved consciousness. I got a glimpse into the consciousness of a paramahamsa, a liberated soul. Some benevolent force had stepped in to raise my concentration when I needed it most. I felt cradled. Completely protected. As strange as this sounds, I felt incredibly safe.

Next, everything just stopped. I somehow wandered out of the club and into the cold night air and empty streets, still thinking that my friends were in the club and being beaten, perhaps even killed. I stood on the street and desperately tried to flag down cars. My drum and I were covered head to toe in blood, so it made sense that no one stopped. Meanwhile, my band had frantically jumped in the van and locked the doors. Tony had turned on the engine and plowed through the roadblock of the bad guys' car. Once the band drove away and did a head count, they realized I wasn't with them, still clueless that I was beaten up.

I realized nobody was going to stop for me, but I kept staggering around looking for help. I must have looked like a monster. I saw a light on in a dirty bus depot. There was a man in a metal-cage booth reading a magazine. I looked him in the eye, and I remember being quite lucid.

"Sir, please call the police, my friends are in big trouble right now."

The man looked up at me. "I'm busy," he said.

"Sir, call the police right now," I said, raising my voice. "Or I'm going to go into that booth, throw you out, and call them myself." I spoke firmly but protectively. The man started the call, and I told him that I was going to hang out in this booth, in case the guys were coming after me. I kneeled in the dirty booth, blood stinging my eyes. I took an inventory of what had just happened to me. I had been hit repeatedly, and my head must have been cracked open.

I was coherent and articulate and felt at total peace—chanting and ready to leave my body. But if I had a concussion, my head would swell. If I fell asleep, I would die in a tamasic, ignorant state, unfocused on my object of meditation. I started to pray. "Oh my Krishna, I wasn't expecting to die tonight! Everything was going so well. The show, the kirtan before the show. It is only the first day of our tour—there is so much more to do. I always knew, and even sang about, how this world is like a dream. We think it's solid, but it fades. And tonight, it is going to fade away for good. My dear Krishna, you gave me a glimpse of what it was like to be God conscious tonight, and it was beautiful. But now I fear my head will swell, I'll fall asleep, and I won't be able to meditate on you. So please, my dear Krishna, if you are going to take me tonight, please take me now, while I am conscious."

I closed my eyes and imagined the most charming picture of Krishna— smiling, with a peacock feather in his hair, wearing yellow garments and holding his bamboo flute. With that dazzling image in my mind I, unfortunately, lived. I say *unfortunately* because it was the only time in my life that I was completely prepared for death.

I was taken to the hospital, a horrific and unsettling experience in itself because of the utter indifference of the staff. After hours of waiting, I was cleaned up and examined. "Nothing's fractured," the doctor said. "There's no concussion. Just minor scrapes. Here's some ibuprofen. Here's a cane. You may need this for a few days. Otherwise, I think you're going to be fine."

I left the hospital and went out to the curb with Henry and K. C. We'd all regrouped after the police arrived. Henry called us a taxi and paid for a nice hotel for us to stay in that night. K. C. sat next to me on the curb, and we waited for the taxi. We were both quiet for a moment.

"The miracle is not that I'm unscathed, or that nothing is broken," I said. "The miracle is that I was taken care of by Krishna as I was about to leave my body. That was magic. I'm not spiritually advanced. I still struggle with all the basics, with controlling my senses and mind, but I was focused and fearless during what I thought were my final moments. You know, there are some yogic practices where you have to control your senses, isolate yourself, move your prana upward, and diligently focus on your third eye. It's a rigid, mechanical way of staying fixed in meditation. Bhakti is different. We just serve and cry out, as a child cries for its mother, and we are taken care of. This tragedy has given me more faith in what we were doing than anything. More than any book, any person, class, or kirtan. I have full faith that I was 100 percent protected, despite my spiritual disqualification."

K. C. put his arm around me. "It's an amazing quality of people practicing bhakti to experience joy and appreciation even in tragic situations," he said. Then we just sat, both deep in thought. After a while, K. C. spoke again. "And the interesting thing, Raghu, is now we're sitting here, all the excitement over, waiting for our taxi, and the real illusion, the real hype of the material world is *now we think we are safe.* What an illusion."

I lay in the hotel room for two days, unable to move. Three days later we played a show in Indianapolis. I kept the cane for a few more weeks, until I could walk without it.

*　*　*

The Buffalo incident brought a new sobriety into my life, a sobriety about life's temporality and how at any moment situations can go from ideal to unreal without warning. It seemed that was an ongoing theme of my life. A lesson I must learn. Therefore, keeping my spiritual identity at the forefront of my life was paramount. I needed to do all my work in this world as though I was in meditation, never forgetting the goal. A mother cow may look like she's fully engaged in eating grass, but she always has an eye out for her calf. Likewise, the endeavoring spiritualist always sees Krishna, or God, in the heart despite engaging in activities in the material sphere. Touring with Shelter around the United States that year became like that. Training myself to be in this world but not of this world. Screaming my head off on stage but singing softer songs of appreciation and kirtan backstage. Standing up tall, being big, and taking up space in front of the crowds but deeply realizing my tiny insignificance in the bigger picture of things. Finding genuine significance in my offering and reconnection to divinity no matter how small. Magic was happening. I was doing the same exact thing I was doing before my dive into spiritual life, but now it was bringing me peace of mind and deeper satisfaction.

On tour, we would often stay with promoters who would put us up at their homes. Generally, they were fans of the band. We were likely a change of pace from other bands, who would drink, party, and maybe even trash the place. We would tell the promoter to invite as many people over to the house as he was comfortable with. Then we'd clean the kitchen spotless and cook a feast of basmati rice, chapatis, dal, curried vegetables, and a sweet. I'd give a class on the *Bhagavad Gita*, and then we'd have a short kirtan and serve the feast. Occasionally, we'd visit a temple or invite the temple devotees to come to our performances.

We'd exhaust ourselves on tour, and then like deciduous trees in winter, we'd hunker down and hibernate into a more traditional monk life either in the ashram or in India.

* * *

I was fascinated by mystics. I had met many in India—and not just the ones who knew the hard sciences, like Ayurveda, Jyotish (Vedic astrology), palmistry, and so on. Those subjects are somewhat mystical, but one can learn them systematically, in the same way one learns auto mechanics. Most people in the West called them quackery or pseudoscience, but in my experience they were incredibly accurate. I've also met people—healers and seers—who use these sciences but perceive things beyond them. They have a mystical gift, or siddhi.

I met a powerful palm reader and visionary once while walking through the streets of Bengal with Porcell. The science of palm reading, or Samudrika

Shastra as it's called in India, is like reading another language. As we walked through the tropical villages, we came upon a humble hut that had a sign in children's writing that said, "Palmistry. One hundred rupees." We looked at each other. Porcell also had a passion for the supernatural and occult, but being street savvy New Yorkers, we didn't trust people just because they hung a sign. Draped in our orange robes, we cautiously approached the shack.

"Are you the palm reader?"

A beautiful man wearing ragged but clean robes and kurta came outside. He had a bold, smiling face that was unshaven and oily but had clean skin. He had perfect teeth and shoulder-length, straight, jet-black hair, which was combed back neatly. His tulasi beads were wrapped in many strands around his neck. "Yes, I am from a family of palm readers. Give me your hand."

I tested him. "Are you a *good* palm reader? I don't mind paying the rupees, but I've met so many charlatans who are trying to make money but are not very good. Before I pay you, tell me something about myself."

He approached me now, skeptical and less enthusiastic if not smug. He gripped my hand, unmoved by my doubt. "You will have three children, you will—"

"No, no, Pandit-ji," I said, cutting him off sharply. "Don't tell me something about my future. You could make up anything. I want to know about my past. Tell me something about my past that only I would know. Then I will pay the rupees."

He nodded again, now annoyed. He looked at my hand up and down, poked at my palm with his index finger, held it sideways, and let it go. "You are a famous musician and have a bad liver."

Whoa, I thought. I had recently been diagnosed with a weak liver by a mystical Ayurvedic healer in New Delhi, and there was no way this village palm reader could possibly know about my musical past. I pulled out one hundred rupees, which he accepted nonchalantly.

Porcell interrupted. "Tell me something about my past, too, Pandit-ji!"

"You, too, are a famous musician." Porcell handed him one hundred rupees as well. And for the next thirty minutes, this insightful older gentleman ripped apart our palms, like he was reading a newspaper—past, present, and future. He told us of our past poor choices and past good fortune. He spoke of tours we had been on. Places we had gone and even romances before we were monks. He spoke of greater success yet to come, but then his face soured, as if he was eating an unripe persimmon.

He looked me in the eye gravely. "But you will get in a tragic car accident. Namaste." Then he quickly turned and went back into his hut, leaving me and Porcell stunned.

"What do you mean 'tragic car accident, namaste'?" I shouted, chasing after him.

"There's nothing I can do. It is in the hand."

"Will I die?" I asked meekly.

"No. No one will die."

I started thinking of all the horrible things that could happen in a car accident without death. Loss of limbs. Crippling disfigurement. Wheelchairs. Burns. The more I thought about it, the more I thought it could be worse than a death sentence.

"What about me, Pandit-ji?" Porcell asked nervously. Will I get into a tragic accident, or just Raghu? Does it look like it's Raghu's problem mainly?"

I looked at Porcell slightly disgusted.

He quickly examined my best friend's hand. "Yes, you too. Quite tragic."

"But how can we change it? How can we change our destiny?" I asked.

"You cannot. But no one will die. Namaste." He spun and retreated into his home.

The strange thing about this incident was that both Porcell and I had heard from less-than-reputable palm readers about a tragic car accident that would happen to us. I thought those prophecies came from lousy palm readers. After hearing it from this master, we started to get slightly nervous. I imagined myself in a passenger seat, with Porcell driving carelessly, looking out the window, crossing double lines, adjusting the cassette player, taking his eyes off the road, or merely dozing off at the wheel. I grew resentful, immediately blaming him in my mind for being so careless and risking our lives, blaming him for what he didn't do yet, if in fact it was even him that was going to be irresponsible.

* * *

In spring 1993, I serendipitously met up with Kaustubha in the stunning countryside of Mayapur, West Bengal. We were surprised to see each other and smiled broadly, bowing to each other to offer respect, then embracing like old friends. We stood speechless for a moment, then blurted out how fortunate we were to be there.

"How did we end up here?" I asked.

"Mercy only. Just a couple of losers from the Lower East Side."

We laughed. The punks ended up in the sacred land of Mayapur. Even Porcell, Steve (our old roadie who lived at the farm), and his new wife, Kate, joined us for a tropical mystical adventure. We, along with a few hundred other devotees from India and around the world, chose Mayapur to attend a special event called Gaura Mandal Parikrama, which roughly translates to walking around to holy places of Sri Chaitanya, the Kirtan Avatar.

It was an incredible ten-day journey through the breathtaking countryside of West Bengal. Tractor carts or bullock carts carried our baggage so we were free to walk while chanting on our beads and singing with two hundred other devotees. The brahmacharis from Mayapur led the *kirtans* and sounded like denizens of a higher planet. They coordinated melodies, or ragas, with certain times of the day, which subtly brought out different emotions in those listening and singing along. We walked through rice paddies and sugarcane groves, which contained clay huts where the harvested canes were cooked down into jaggery, a sweetener and medicine because of its high mineral content. Sometimes we'd cross rivers in multiple boats piloted by local boatmen who'd been waiting for us to arrive. Coconut and date palms lined the roads, as did mango and jackfruit trees.

We would walk to a holy place while one of the senior swamis would explain its significance. Hawkers selling coconuts would approach us, deftly wielding machetes to pop the coconuts' tops and make a large goblet of sorts. After spending fifteen or twenty minutes at a divine place, we'd continue our walking and singing journey until the next place. Around 1 p.m. we'd stop at a shaded school, ashram, or orchard, where a crew of Mayapur monks were setting up an incredible Bengali feast for us. Rice, fried potato, green spinach, bitter gourd, bitter melon fried in ghee, and banana flower were some of the dishes I could identify. At night there were massive communal tents for men and women. This was like a Krishna-conscious Boy Scout jamboree! Kaustubha and I chose not to sleep in the massive tent. We set up mosquito nets separate from everyone and simply reclined on top of our sleeping bags—the tropical heat was enough to keep us warm.

One night, while observing the stars, Kaustubha started talking. "Christopher Columbus was looking for shorter trade routes to India to acquire the land's wealth in spices, gold, and silks that the Romans and Greeks spoke of, but not only did he miss his destination, he missed out on the real wealth of India. The knowledge. The wisdom. He blew it." We laughed.

"It was the same time Ponce de León was looking for the fountain of youth!" I said. "It's here! It's overcoming old age by understanding that we are spirit, that we don't die, that the bodily conception is like a dream, like a mirage. Both of these guys were in America five hundred years ago, the same time Chaitanya was resurrecting bhakti in India! Bhakti is the real fountain of youth!"

The next day, we crossed the Ganges in a small wooden boat that seemed like it would sink with so many devotees crammed onto it. When we realized there was going to be a wait for the other boats to get across, Kaustubha motioned to me to come to the riverbank.

"Let's do our sacred bath," he said.

I smiled, and we used our cotton turban cloth, wrapping it around the waist as a simple bathing suit. Bowing down, we offered the following prayer:

> O Ganges! Take away my diseases, sorrows,
> difficulties, sins, and wrong attitudes. You are
> the essence of the three worlds, and you are like
> a necklace around the earth. O goddess! You
> alone are my refuge in this samsara.

Then we bowed down on the riverbank, grabbed a palmful of water, and offered it to the Ganges. The water dripped from our palms back into the river itself. We submerged ourselves in the cool water under the hot sun, feeling like we had entered the spiritual realm. The Ganges was magic. This experience was much different than my experience in Kolkata. I had become a different person since my first trip to India. I was tangibly transforming. It was exciting. My thoughts were different, my actions were different, my desires were different . . . I was different.

Kaustubha and I sat on the riverbank and offered prayers for all the punks and hardcore friends of ours who had inspired us on our spiritual journey on the Lower East Side. Somehow, they were tagged by God to speak to us, and we felt indebted.

*   *   *

I journeyed to southern India, where I fasted on water for ten days. I went in search of alternative healers, not necessarily for spiritual benefit, but just to fulfill a passion for health and vitality. I knew India was a treasure trove of all types of physical and metaphysical mysteries. I knew there were pranayamas, yogic breathing techniques, that helped you become healthy, connect with God, and develop mystic powers. I was always interested in the esoteric pranayamas, but I knew they weren't taught in Western yoga books. I was aware that practicing pranayama inappropriately could affect the mind in a bad way, leading to stroke, dementia, and so on. In Ayurvedic medicine, the body's prana, or life airs, control thinking, breathing, evacuating, sneezing, giving birth, and more, and when they are out of alignment, they can cause unforeseen health issues. My study of pranayama had been the basics—ujjayi, nadi shodana, bhastrika, and kapalabhati—which most yogis know. The basics did benefit you because our culture is filled with wrong breathing—mouth breathing, shallow breathing, unconscious breathing. The retention and movement of the prana in a regulated way can also have a mystical, spiritual effect that is not often talked about. After all, the yoga system is essentially a strategy to control the mind, move the prana, and ultimately connect with the divine.

In my travels to South India, I came across a young Ayurvedic doctor named Vikram-ji. I was curious to meet him and ask him for some insight into the more esoteric pranayamas. He dressed traditionally in a South Indian dhoti and beautiful rudraksha beads and wore sacred clay markings on his body and forehead. He was pencil thin, had perfect teeth, and could have been a model if he was living in the United States. Like many Ayurvedic doctors, he was also an astrologer. The idea was that to understand a person's health, you didn't look at only their present body—you looked at their planets and what astrological period they were in, as this also affected health. If a person had a malefic planet at a certain time in their life, no health regimen could heal them. The ailment would go away in due time as the person came into a new astrological period.

Vikram-ji had a good reputation. While I waited in line to see him, I sat outside under the shade of a neem tree. The twigs of the neem tree are the traditional toothbrushes of India. The toothbrush as we know it wasn't invented until the 1800s, but ancient cultures around the globe used to chew sticks, often from bitter or astringent plants such as the neem tree. They'd chew one end until it became frayed and use the other side as a toothpick. They are antibacterial and help keep gums healthy. These are still used in India and among conservative followers of Vedic culture who see the modern toothbrush as unclean. I picked up some twigs to save for later brushing. Then I picked up some leaves and chewed them (they are bitter) because they are considered medicinal, helping with digestion, stomach disorders, fever, and diseases of the gums, heart, and blood vessels. They could even keep mosquitoes away.

Look at this beautiful tree, I thought. *Providing shade, toothbrushes, and medicine. We are so taken care of in this world. Nature has provided everything for us. It proves to me how the universe provides what we need and our dependence on artificial substitutes that make others wealthy not only harm us but also our very planet. Simple living. Keep it simple.*

As the people sitting in front of me went to see the doctor, I sat chanting on my mala. I also kept sacred sounds in my head. I sat peacefully, running my fingers over the tulasi beads.

Finally, when it was my turn, Vikram-ji looked at me. Everyone had left the doctor's open-air office. Before I got up, he looked at me as if he was looking inside of me. "You're not here because you're sick. You want secret pranayamas."

I was shocked by his deliberate and insightful reading of my mind—and how matter-of-fact he was about it.

"I am knowing secret pranayamas, but I cannot give without my guru's permission. I will see him tonight, and I will ask him. Come again tomorrow."

Before I left, I wanted to know more about him. He told me about his lineage and how he also practiced siddhi medicine, which involved a monk sitting in meditation and getting various herbal formulas from higher beings in astral planes. There are many people in India who are not doctors but are from a siddhi family lineage. Usually, the story went that their ancestors worshiped particular demigods or God, and they were given mantras, herbs, and rituals to follow for curing one specific ailment. Then they passed the knowledge down to their children and so on for many generations. On this same trip, Porcell was healed of jaundice by one of these siddhis within three or four days, something that usually took up to six months.

I asked Vikram-ji if he was married, and he said yes but that they do not live together. "I'm working and sending money back to her," he said. "She is in our village with our family." I asked if he had children. His reply shocked me. "I do not. But some people in my tradition have children, and if they are boys, they will give them to the ashram to be raised by the monks."

"You're kidding. Why would anyone do that?" I replied, borderline upset.

"Seeing how you are dressed," he said, "I thought you'd understand. To cultivate detachment." He smiled and assured me that the young boys were loved and got the best training in metaphysics, healing, yoga, and brahmachari life.

"But they're *your* children?" I asked, finding it hard to understand from my Western perspective.

"Yes. It is a difficult practice. It forces us to deeply understand we own nothing in this world. Even the child that comes from our womb and seed. You are a brahmachari. You must understand the value in detachment."

I nodded, not wanting to seem fake, but the practice was still hard to digest.

"As attached as we are to home and family, we own nothing. They are not ours. We must love. But it's only for a few years. Then we lose all that we love. This is the way of material nature, Raghunath. It takes from us all that we love."

I thought of my father's death and how correct and wise this young doctor was.

I was torn between the idea of detachment and being just plain irresponsible. But I wanted to be open-minded to different cultures and ways of living, especially with these otherworldly people I'd met on my journey. I tended to think I had all the answers and that my way was the right way and the only way. This type of thinking cheated me out of an objective education. At the same time, it seemed unnatural to voluntarily give away children even if they will be loved and cared for.

I thought deeply. Whether we gave away a child or not, the doctor was right. There is nothing we can hold on to in this material world. All we can do is love for a few days or decades.

*   *   *

I returned the next day to see Vikram-ji. I wanted the secret pranayamas. When I got to see the young doctor, he said, "I have spoken to my guru. He will not allow me to teach you."

I was crestfallen.

"But he will teach you personally."

"You're kidding. Where does he live?"

"He lives in a cave, but you cannot visit him there. He will come here tomorrow morning. Meet us upstairs in the ashram at 5 a.m."

In the past, many mystics, sadhus, and spiritual recluses lived in caves. Caves were free. No rent. These people were also beggars and went to homes for their daily food. Householders would give them a chapati or some rice and dal, and in this way they were outside of the matrix of material pursuits and could focus on spiritual or mystic yogic practices. If they were doing it right, the traditional way, poverty came from a voluntary choice to focus their energy on spiritual topics. This was why—and this is true even today—such people were given the highest respect in Indian society. Their detachment, introspection, and deep spiritual study kept them impartial and learned. They were philosophical educators who led by example. I wanted to go to the cave of the doctor's guru, but I was happy he was coming in the morning.

Before sunrise, I went to the ashram and sat cross-legged on a kusha, or a traditional prayer mat, and started my japa there. Vikram-ji came in, looking gorgeous as usual, with his morning shawl, slick hair, and bright yellow dhoti. An elderly man followed in an orange dhoti and a plain, thick, wool chadar, resembling a horse blanket, wrapped around his body and head. Only his charming face showed. He was unshaven, and I noticed his feet. They were like shoes, leathery and thick from walking barefoot for decades perhaps. He had a belly, but that's the beauty of a dhoti—it can be loosened. One size fits all. He said something in Malayalam, the local language, to his young disciple.

"He wants to know why you want to learn these pranayamas," Vikram-ji said, translating for me. The guru stood earnestly.

I was put on the spot. I didn't want to say, "Because I thought it would be cool." Instead, I replied, "I practice bhakti yoga, and therefore whatever I learn I want to use in the service of Bhagavan."

He translated what I said to the guru, who nodded in agreement, as if I had passed the test. He instructed me on breathing techniques, mudras, retention techniques, and a mantra. "Without the mantra you will not get full benefit," Vikram-ji said.

I nodded, understanding the potency of mantras and continued our practices. Then, after Vikram-ji had performed the techniques for about fifteen minutes in front of his guru, he came over and swiftly slapped me on the third eye. This is called the shaktipata, or the transfer of shakti. It was as if an electric current went through me, an energetic buzz I'd never felt before, like the first time I had an orgasm. He made me continue the breathing techniques for a while and made sure I was accomplished in them. Then he nodded, I bowed, and he left.

I continued with this meditation practice for some time. It was powerful, both physically and psychically. I felt a deep relaxation within my body and a calm over my consciousness. I felt as if it was igniting and awakening something inside of me. I also found it improved my overall health, but that was the side benefit—this was primarily a spiritual practice. I felt detachment from the pain of the world, like I wasn't part of this world. It took me to places where there was no me any longer. No relationships. No family. No pain. No heartbreak. No me.

But I was torn. The problem was that the mantras I was given were for impersonalists. Many, if not most, in this culture accept that there is a higher power, but they give that energy an impersonal name, such as Brahman. But the mantras that resonated the most with me were personal and used primary names of God—Bala Gopal, Krishna, Govinda, Rama, and so on. Although I understood that the impersonal aspects of God are real, I had a strong attachment to the personal features of divinity. I felt like the impersonal mantras were taking me away from sweet Krishna, whom I had grown to cherish in my heart. After a while, I knew I couldn't continue. I knew it was not my path.

*   *   *

I headed back to northern India, back to Vrindavan. It was cold, dark, and damp at 6 a.m., and I was reading from a tattered old book called the *Upadeshamrita,* or *The Nectar of Instruction.* According to the book, there were six principles favorable to bhakti yoga, and the first three really caught my attention. They almost sounded *too* simple: (1) being enthusiastic, (2) endeavoring with confidence, and (3) being patient. These could just as likely be found in a business or self-help book. But I spent the day saying and reading them, thinking of how to apply them on my journey. They immediately turned out to be useful.

One day, I was heading toward the sacred lakes of Radha Kunda and Shyama Kunda, where I planned to do parikrama. On my first trip to India, I did parikrama by walking around the holy town of Vrindavan each day, but you can do parikrama around holy hills, a holy forest, or even a holy tree. Sometimes people, in a gesture of intense devotion, hold a rock in their hand and bow down flat on the ground with their arms extended. This is called dandavat, or full prostration. Then they drop the stone where their hands are, push themselves up, and step to the stone. They pick it up and do it again and again and again, moving gradually around the sacred object.

I was intrigued and attracted to this concept of full-contact prayer. I knew I had to do it. I started small with a minor dandavat (which means "falling like a stick") parikrama around the sacred lakes. I was told by an experienced devotee that it should take three to four hours to complete. *Not bad. I can do this!* I thought.

The two lakes are in the center of a small village that is also called Radha Kunda. All the saints, swamis, and sacred literature say that this village was one of the most intimate places for Krishna bhakti. It is said that those who live on the banks of Radha Kunda are liberated souls, that the dust on the ground is sacred, and that the water in these lakes is liquid love. Even the animals here—the bugs, dogs, monkeys, and pigs—are exalted beings. It's their last life, and they are burning off some karma before emancipation from this world.

The sacred literature recommended that you didn't see this place with ordinary vision. It was a vortex to another dimension, and what appeared ordinary was actually extraordinary. I struggled with this. My material vision tried to assess the village. Yes, it had a charm to it, especially on this peaceful early morning with only the sound of sweet *kirtan*s from the ashrams bordering the sacred lakes. But it was not what by Western standards would be called pristine.

I prayed to suspend my material vision and see this place for what it was: a transcendental realm of extraordinary beings who had the great fortune to reside there. I would resist critiquing or criticizing any material contamination I might see. That was my mantra: *Suspend your material vision. See this village through the eyes of the sacred literature and the saints.*

With a prayerful mind on that early morning, I picked up a stone the size of a golf ball to mark my spot and bowed down on that quiet, narrow lane, extending my hands in full prostration. Immediately, three kids on bicycles zipped by carelessly, nearly running over my fingers. I went from peaceful to pissed in a matter of seconds.

I'm lying on the road, I thought, feeling full of dread and slightly disturbed. *What do I expect?*

Three men were shooting the breeze in the street, taking up most of the narrow path. I was lying on the ground next to their feet, religiously bowing down and getting up. They didn't even look at me, or move for that matter. It was embarrassing, truthfully. These guys weren't talking about anything spiritual. They were just talking, and I was some dopey white guy with a robe lying down on the street. I felt so awkward.

There was a poor villager ahead of me sweeping the streets with a jharu, a homemade broom made from bound grasses or reeds. I felt fortunate that he was there, in essence cleaning the street for me, but I was acutely aware of all the dust kicked up and how that can affect one's lungs. I knew what a devotee might have been thinking, *This is the dust of the feet of great souls, the sacred dust of animals, saints, and sages.*

But I wasn't thinking that. I wasn't thinking of my mantra either. I had a new mantra that went something like this: *Am I going to get emphysema from this dust? I'm going to get emphysema from this dust. I know it. I'm going to get emphysema. God knows what's in this dust. Particles of dirt, or course, and maybe specks of feces.*

My mind spun more out of control. *What the hell am I doing? What am I trying to prove? Does this act make me more spiritual, or am I just an idiot?"* It was amazing how fast I could go from spiritual consciousness to total maya.

I continued down the narrow path, with the sacred pond Radha Kunda sparkling in the morning sun. I had to keep moving if I was going to beat the heat. When it gets hot, it gets very hot very quickly, and the stone path and pavement I was bowing down upon would heat up like a pizza oven.

I kept moving. Up and down bowing. Up and down bowing. It was like doing push-ups. Even though I was bowing, I tried not to put my face near the ground, because of the emphysema, TB, and malaria mantras running through my head.

This is bad, I thought. I needed an attitude adjustment and a new mantra. I started chanting in my head, *O Radha and Krishna, please direct me. Please guide me.* Up and down. Bowing. Up and down. Move the rock forward. *I am your servant. What would you like from me in this short life, my Lord? Please direct me.* That was a great mantra, and I did that for fifteen minutes. Up and down. Move the rock. *Jai Sri Krishna! Jai Sri Radhey! Jai Sri Krishna! Jai Sri Radhey! Suspend my material vision! See through the eyes of the saints! I am a servant of the great souls.*

As I stood up, I looked ahead and noticed a mother shaving her young child's head. She was throwing the hair into the street, directly onto the path ahead of me.

Oh Krishna! I'm going to get sick, I thought. *Where's that sweeper? I hope he gets that hair up before I reach it. I'm in a bad headspace again. Jai Sri Krishna! Jai Sri Radhey!* I try to refocus, recalibrate. *Holy place. Holy people. Spiritual vortex. Sacred lake. Liquid love!*

I continued on, skillfully dodging the hair in the process of my bowing and getting up. Every time I stood, I was less in prayer and more in scout mode. What was ahead of me on the path? Twenty feet further, I noticed the pavement was wet across the width of the path. Small puddles were visible, too. *What kind of water is in that puddle? What made that area wet?* It could have been spilled holy water or urine from one of the wandering goats. Or maybe somebody had dropped a pot of tea. It could have been anything.

I was starting to lose my mind in addition to my focused, clear, blissful state. Then I heard a beautiful kirtan in the distance. It lightened my heart and cleared my head. The sun started to warm me at the perfect temperature. I passed the subji market, where a bunch of ladies sold fresh vegetables spread out on colorful cotton blankets. I could smell the fragrance of cut papayas, tangerines, and nimbus, tiny lemons. The phool wallahs were selling fragrant flower garlands of marigolds, roses, and jasmines. Their intoxicating perfume invigorated my spirit and gave my senses a reprieve from my mental demons. Up and down. Up and down.

My dear Radha and Krishna, how can I serve you in this short life? I thought. *I'm grateful. I'm blessed. I'm grateful. I'm grateful for all the teachers in my life. Thank you.* I started running through a list of teachers and messengers that had been sent to me, including Harley Flanagan, the teenage gang leader who first explained bhakti to me. I realized that messengers had always been sent to me, but sometimes I simply couldn't and wouldn't hear from them. God was always trying to reclaim us. But we missed out on the magic. We were all magical, spiritual beings, but we had developed a love affair with the matter of the world, like a fish obsessed with the baited hook. I pictured every face and name that had assisted me on my spiritual path, from the local teachers in Vrindavan to the monks I met along the way to my band members to my parents. *I'm grateful. I'm blessed. I'm honored to be here,* I prayed. *Hare Krishna. Jai Sri Radhey. Jai Sri Krishna.*

I lay down, and a big, wet pig scampered by. *Oh my God. Oh my Krishna!* Pigs in India are grotesque, often sleeping in the open sewers. This one was soaking wet with sewer water all over him. He was probably splattering raw sewage right on my path. *Emphysema. Dengue fever. Leprosy. Elephantiasis.* I started listing any disease that came to my spinning mind.

A few children dressed like Oliver Twist were selling hardened clay from the bottom of the lake used for tilaka. They tried to sell me some. I was in prayer-meets-freakout mode, so I said nothing and continued forward.

This went on for almost two hours. Up and down. Deep prayer but distracted. Self-conscious. Inspired. Worried. Exuberant. A confused assortment of all the emotions. There was something beautifully exhausting in this full-contact prayer. I was sweating and sore but exhilarated from all the ups and downs. It cleared my head. I started getting a workout high, an endorphin rush.

I started praying out loud, singing "Sri Krishna Govinda, Hari Murari, Hey Natha Narayana, Vasudeva!" People looked at me, smiled. It was a holy village, so somebody chanting and screaming the names of God out loud was business as usual. I stood up, holding my stone, but my enthusiasm came to a dead stop. About four meters ahead, a pack of monkeys blocked my path. These monkeys can get rough, and they're fearless. I continued cautiously. Up and down. Push up. Stand, pray. Down. Extend my rock and move forward.

Please back up, monkeys, I thought. I noticed some of the monkeys *had* moved to the side, making room for me. Then all moved, except one. One lone monkey blocked the path, the biggest of them all. And gnarly looking. He was missing a paw and had a scarred face and protruding tooth, all of which made him look like a savage, slightly unhinged pirate.

I kept going. I bowed, and I remembered something I'd read about this place. Every living being in this place was a great sage who had died and had a little karma left to burn in this incarnation. This was their last life. These weren't ferocious monkeys. These were pure souls, more evolved than me. The pirate monkey was a great sage in a previous life. These are holy people, merely polishing and fine-tuning themselves on their journey home!

I'm blessed and fortunate to be here. I'm the one who doesn't belong, I thought. *These living beings . . . all of them are my prabhus, my masters who have traveled the soul's journey for many lifetimes and are standing on the precipice of perfection.*

I became enthusiastic, just as the book I was reading said I should be. New mantra: *Enthusiasm, confidence, patience!* Instead of avoiding him, I went full speed ahead toward that pirate monkey with a smile on my face, imagining how I could touch the sacred lotuslike feet of any of these saintly monkeys. I extended my hand, reaching for them, practically chasing them, but with gentle, fearless movement. I caught one of the slower ones and rubbed his foot dust onto my forehead. The rest, including the pirate monkey, scampered out of my way when they saw how fearless and confident I was.

Next came four or five goats herded by a teen. I grabbed the little hoof of the goat and touched my head to it. "This is no ordinary being," I said out loud. "This is a transcendental being in a goat body! Give me your mercy, Goat!" The other goats scampered away. The little boy looked at me strangely. Then, while lying prostrate on the ground, I touched *his* feet. The boy scampered away with his small herd, smiling at my insanity but understanding the gesture and intention as sincere.

Twenty or so old men from the Manipur temple came by, like a ragtag marching band, melodiously chanting the *Mahamantra*. They saw my devotion and excitement and cheered me on. I dove for their transcendental feet. They dodged my grip, but I persisted. "Ashirvat dedjie!" I yelled. "Give me your mercy!" In a frenzy I started zipping down the path—up, down, up, down, reaching for feet. Loudly chanting names of Radha and Krishna.

I was speaking like a madman possessed by spirit. I turned the corner for the final stretch. My body and clothes were very dirty, stained by the dust and dirt and the mystery puddles. My spirits were high. Five beggar women were next on my radar to touch their lotuslike feet.

"The lowest part of *their* body I consider to be incredibly sacred," I repeated as I moved between the women. I felt a warmth and love in my heart for every being I saw. I started to develop the genuine vision that the earth I was bowing to was filled with holy dust. I went down to bow, and I decided to stay down and appreciate all the saints that had walked on this path. "Thank you. Thank you. Thank you."

Exhausted but euphoric, I completed my full circle around the village in only three hours.

Wouldn't it be wonderful if at every moment I could have deep appreciation for all beings and see them with incredible dignity and treat them all as exalted souls? I immediately understood the simple but profound lesson to look past the shells of people and animals and see them for what they are. Nobody and nothing is ordinary. Everyone and everything is extraordinary. I remembered the three principles from the *Upadeshamrita* that I had been studying: (1) being enthusiastic, (2) endeavoring with confidence, (3) being patient.

I wrote the following in my journal: "These three alone can change my entire existence on earth."

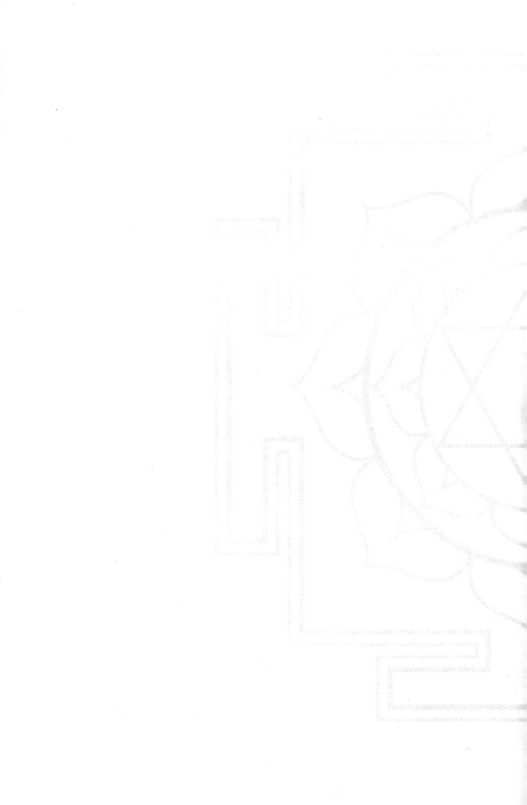

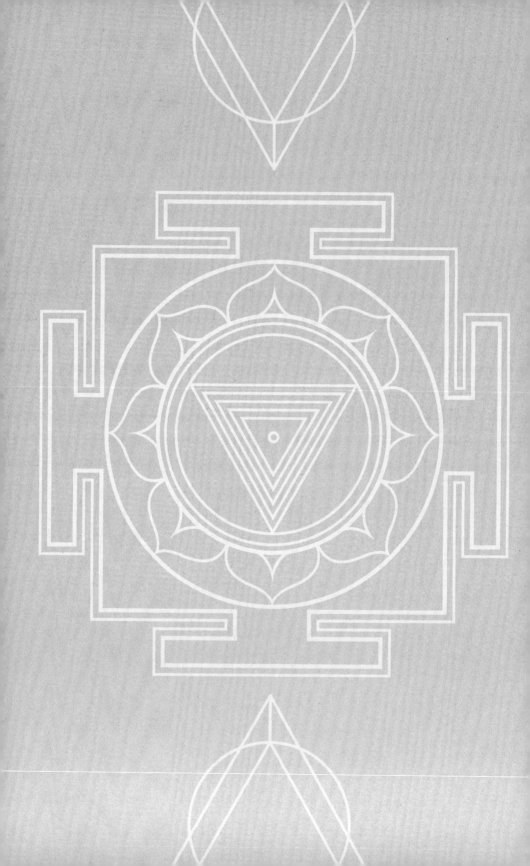

CHAPTER 11

LIFE AFTER THE ASHRAM

Kaustubha's guru, Goswami Maharaj, was a senior monk and guru whom I loved. He had taken care of me since I first entered the ashram and taught me so many facets of spiritual culture. The word guru can also mean "heavy," and Goswami Maharaj could be just that. He had the ability to crush the false ego with a few sharp words. Sometimes he would raise his voice, and his chastisements could be devastating, but he always knew how to make you feel incredibly loved as well.

This fierce love helped me grow out of my ego. In the same way a surgeon uses a scalpel to get into the body to repair it and thus heal the person, Goswami Maharaj would chop into my narcissism, ignorance, and arrogance, and he taught me how to be a man. He became yet another wise, strong, and loving father figure to me.

It was 1994, and the year was wrapping up. I had lived in the ashrams for six years. Goswami Maharaj called me into his room one day and asked me if I ever thought about getting married. I was twenty-eight years old. I enjoyed being a monk. He noticed that our band was getting bigger and that required me to be out in the world more and more.

"If you're thinking about it at all, or thinking about being a father, you may want to leave the life of being a brahmachari and become a dutiful householder. After all, I've seen monks hang in there longer than they should have. It's not good, Raghunath. They can lose touch with the material world and can't ever figure out how to maintain a family."

I thought leaving the ashram was a smart choice. Become a dutiful householder. Shelter was getting bigger. We got signed to Roadrunner Records, a large international record label that had an office in New York. The band had moved to the ashram in Brooklyn to be closer to the label, which was investing a lot in Shelter. We were going to record an album, and Roadrunner was planning a world tour.

"Raghunath, living outside an ashram will give you some freedom, but with that freedom is always a responsibility," said Goswami Maharaj one day. "Being out in the world and trying not to get swept away by the world, well, that's a slippery slope. A strong daily spiritual sadhana can protect you."

"Like what?"

"Spend quality time chanting japa and reading the *Srimad Bhagavatam*. Continue to spend time in holy places and going to India. Don't get proud of any of your success. Material success can ruin your life and your intelligence. See all success as Krishna's mercy upon you and offer it back to Him with love and gratitude."

I took Goswami Maharaj's advice to heart, and although I lived in the ashram for six months more, I started entering a new phase of life. The day after our conversation, I took off my sadhu's saffron robes and put on white robes with dignity, signifying the next stage. How to be in the world but not of it. It was a tricky transition. How to be close to the water's edge without getting wet. After all, a lot of cultural changes had happened in the world, whereas I had been leading a somewhat cloistered life since 1988. Living outside the ashram proved to be a balancing act despite all the study and time spent in the ashram.

We released our album, called *Mantra*, on CD. On the cover we put the benevolent Ganga Devi, the goddess of the sacred Ganges River, where I'd had many profound realizations. It is said that to anyone who simply bathes in her water, she awards material success, freedom from pain, and most of all, pure devotion to Krishna.

*   *   *

In 1996, I jumped into a taxicab to take me from the record company office to the hotel to meet the band. It had been less than a year since I'd given up monk life. As part of our world tour, we were in Brazil, where the label had thoroughly set up the record for maximum success. I could feel Shelter's popularity growing. It felt good to be in the tropical heat and humidity with the fragrances of nag champa and magnolia mixed with the fragrances of fresh-fruit markets. Even in the bustling city of São Paulo, these scents were apparent. I was excited to be there and excited for this fast-paced tour that would take me to all of Brazil's major cities, as well as Buenos Aires, Argentina, and Bogotá, Colombia.

The cab driver was blasting the radio, which I didn't mind, as it was sort of an interesting cultural experience hearing both the songs and advertisements from a foreign country. But then our song "Here We Go" from our new CD came on the radio. *Weird? Coincidence?* I thought. Was this a *local* radio station? A small university station, like the ones at home that occasionally played our music on obscure punk college radio shows? Did the station have something to do with the record company? We were on the same record label as the internationally massively influential Brazilian metal band Sepultura. Did the record company have so much influence over the local radio station that they'd be playing our song?

I asked the driver, "Is this a local radio station?

He smiled. "No, no! This is TransAmerica radio. The biggest station in our nation. This is the most famous radio station in all of Brazil."

He dropped me off at the hotel. The band was there and met me in astonishment. Our drummer, Roy, spoke first. "Raghu, you're never going to believe what happened. We were in the mall just looking around and some kids said, 'Hey it's Shelter!' and all of a sudden we were surrounded by kids coming in all directions asking for autographs, pieces of our clothing, asking us to write on their bodies or clothing. Tons of kids! It was so weird!"

Our bass player, Franklin, chimed in. "I'm thinking we may be bigger here than we realize."

The band was right. We found out that we had three songs in high rotation on TransAmerica radio, as well as dozens of regional radio stations around South America. MTV Brazil had been playing our video constantly and was asking us to come on for an interview. TransAmerica radio invited us to play live on the air. All of this attention in the press and media made the shows sell out in big venues and put us on an exhausting but exhilarating whirlwind tour around the nation, from Belém to Curitiba.

Before we started playing, we did a series of interviews. Our promoters picked us up in a van along with a carful of bodyguards, drove us from the airport, and swiftly delivered us to the local temple in Rio de Janeiro for a press conference. Interviewers, reporters, and film crews from radio stations and newspapers were waiting patiently for our arrival. We spent the night at a gorgeous hotel on Ipanema Beach. I rose early and did pranayama on the beach. Next, I sat in one place for two hours to chant sixteen rounds of japa. It kept me balanced. Distress, loss, heartbreak, and anxiety aren't the only factors that could throw me off my spiritual trajectory. Success, fame, and public validation could do it, too. Chanting the sacred mantras, especially the holy name, protected me from the influence of the ego and the arrogance that came with good fortune. I also decided on this trip to add chanting a chapter of the *Bhagavad Gita* in Sanskrit and English as a morning ritual while on tour, which turned out to be powerful.

That day, after I finished chanting chapter 9 of the *Gita*, the sun was just rising. I knew the band was in the hotel, perhaps a little jet-lagged. I wanted to bathe in the ocean before diving into a tropical fruit breakfast, but nobody was on the beach and the waves were massive. I was a little intimidated. However, I reflected on Ayurvedic teachings about the power of morning bathing in sun and salt water before eating. I was inspired, so I ran back to the hotel to get my bathing suit and towel and to see if anyone else was awake yet. Bossa nova played in the hotel restaurant. The band members were all asleep, but Paulo, our Brazilian press agent and liaison from the record company, was downstairs eating some toast and sliced fruit.

Paulo was sweet and lovable and arranged all my interviews. It didn't take much for me to convince him to go for a walk on the beach with me.

"Let's go in the water and swim a little," I said.

"These waves are too big for me, Raghu. I'm not sure about it."

I urged him to go in for a refreshing morning bath. I spoke about the power of salt water and morning sun. I also mentioned that the waves were breaking far out and we could stay in the shallow water.

My persuasion worked, and soon, under that hot morning tropical sun, we were feeling the refreshing salt water of the South Atlantic Ocean on our skin. It was as though we had the entire ocean to ourselves as the city slept in. I submerged myself and laughed like a child in the waves with Paulo. What a perfect morning! What a perfect day, and it wasn't even 8 a.m.! Besides being in the present moment and carving time for wholesome sadhana and self-care, I was also hopeful for the tour, which was starting the next day. After dunking myself in and out of the refreshing water a few more times, I noticed that I didn't see Paulo any longer. Then I saw only his face, appearing like an island through the top of the water's surface.

"Help me, I'm drowning," he said softly but urgently. "I have a severe cramp. Please help me, I'm drowning." He wasn't far out, but the water was choppy, and he was in a bit over his head. I thought maybe he was joking.

Then the surf covered his face, and he spouted up water from his mouth like the blowhole of a whale. "Help me!" he said more loudly. "Please help me! I have a cramp and I'm drowning!"

I was caught off guard by this sudden turn—from playful frolicking to potential tragedy. I swam over, still not sure if he was being serious or not.

"Paulo, are you okay?"

"Help me!" he said loudly. "I'm drowning! Help me!"

As I got closer to him, I did exactly what lifeguards teach *not* to do: I approached from the front. Never approach a drowning person from the front. He grabbed me—out of instinct and desperation—digging his nails into my skin and forcing my head underwater. I began choking on the salty water entering my mouth. I struggled desperately. My feet hit the ocean floor as he climbed on top of me. I sprang to the surface.

"Paulo!" I screamed.

He was frantic. "Help! Help me!"

He again gripped me, scratching me, clawing at me, and pulling me under the water. I choked and coughed, but I was still more concerned with Paulo, as I had never heard a friend calling out for his life. A local passerby ran into the water, grabbed Paulo, and dragged him out, giving him aid and comfort at the eleventh hour. In my attempt to save Paulo, I didn't realize I was now in a precarious position myself. A riptide current threatened to drag me deeper into the ocean. I was already exhausted from fighting Paulo off me. I had drunk a lot of salt water from being held underwater. Everything instantly switched, and I realized that I was now the one in need. I saw Paulo far in the distance, lying on the beach with the man by his side. Panic set in. Now I was helpless! I started to plead, abandoning all modesty. "Help me! Help me!" I screamed out.

They didn't see or hear me. Before I shouted my third petition for help, I was nailed by a wave, which spun me underwater, tossing and tumbling me. I lost all sense of which direction to swim to get to the surface. I finally surfaced. But as soon as I could inhale, another wave nailed me. I was choking and coughing and exhausted. I tried my best to keep my cool as the heavy water held me under its surface. When I finally was buoyed upward, the riptide dragged me so far past the waves into the ocean it was almost laughable. I was so far from the shore, already without energy, and still coughing water out of my mouth.

I tried to apply some yoga techniques. *I gotta not panic*, I thought. *I've gotta control my mind or else it will become my enemy. I have to breathe. I have to relax. I have to stay afloat and scream for some passersby for any being to hear me and help.*

I calmed myself slightly, caught some air, and screamed at the top of my lungs, relinquishing any ego or pride. "Help me, I'm drowning!"

A quietude came over me. *Nobody can hear you, Raghunath*, I gravely told myself. *You're too far from the shore at this point. You need divine intervention. You're going to have to call out to God. Only God can help you now.* I regained my composure and screamed at the top of my waterlogged lungs. "Oh Krishna, help me, I'm drowning!"

Nothing.

Raghu, no people are going to help you, I thought. *Krishna's not going to help you. You are going to die. And people die and have died like this every day throughout history. Accidents. Careless choices. Riptides. You are not special. You are not a rock star. You are just a statistic. An obituary in a Rio de Janeiro newspaper that will be skimmed over and discarded. You just weren't expecting* this *to be the day.*

I lamented that we came all the way to Brazil and didn't play one show. It seemed like a waste. Then my study of Vedic texts started challenging that thought. *Yep, that's material existence*, I thought. *Unfulfilled material expectations and death and loss are sneaking up right behind us, as a lion stalks a deer. You knew this, Raghunath. Don't get too excited about material success. It can end in a moment.*

I felt my increasing weakness yet still floated helplessly.

None of my bandmates will know where I was or what happened to me, I thought. *I didn't say goodbye to anyone! My mother doesn't know where I am at all! My death will be a mystery to her. I never thanked her for all she has done for me! But this is how it happens, I suppose. When you least expect it. When you're filled with hope. When you have a plan. Before you have closure with the world, say a goodbye, or make a public statement. Today is that day for me.*

Then a final thought came to mind. *At least I woke up early today, sat and chanted for two hours, and read the* Bhagavad Gita. *At least I did that today!*

I had read of people leaving this world in deep transcendental consciousness. Fear, anxiety, and desperation were not present. They were happy in understanding not only that they cannot die but that life without the burden of the body would be even more blissful. For those in material bondage like me, the body was merely a heavy yet temperamental piece of luggage the soul carried around. It tended to break down, get diseased, age hideously, smell. The subtle body of the conditioned soul often felt mental anguish, false hope, and unfulfilled desire—or, stewed in resentment, unable to forgive.

Once the bodily actions of the consciousness were purified, the great souls remained in this world but not of this world. These mahatmas shed the body with no lamentation, just as someone peels off a heavy coat and layers of clothes when stepping into their home. They saw the body for what it was, a gift from material nature to live out its material desires, but it became a gift they outgrew. I lamented that I had not outgrown my material desires, even with all my talk, lyrics, and interviews about the importance of our spiritual pursuit. I lamented that I wasn't more evolved. More serious. More connected internally and more kind externally. I lamented that, although I made an endeavor, I had not reached a perfected state of being. I hadn't become a sage. I would have to take birth again and spin the wheel of fortune, hoping to get the opportunity for somebody to put me back on the path.

I prayed with all sincerity while still desperately trying to tread water. "Oh Lord Krishna, I was not expecting to die today, but today you chose to take me. I relinquish my desire to cling to this body. But, sweet Krishna, I'm still impure. I know this. I only ask you to please let me take birth in a family that sincerely practices bhakti yoga, and I pray to take full advantage of such good fortune."

At that point I gave up resisting. I accepted the loss of my body to the powerful and superior ocean, and I felt relieved from my physical struggle. I gave my life to God's hands and surrendered, praying to Him to take me. I uttered a mantra to assist my passing: "Jaya Sri Krishna Chaitanya, Prabhu Nityananda, Sri Advaita, Gadadhara, Srivasadi Gaura Bhakta Vrinda."

Water entered my mouth, the salt burned my throat and stomach, my arms stopped flailing, and I submerged. Some piece of innate will flapped my arms so I'd surface again. I saw a local boy, about twelve years old, coming to save me while paddling fiercely on a longboard. I continued chanting, not knowing if I'd make it out or not by the time he got to me.

But he made it. I lived. This near-death experience helped me stay sober-minded amid the so-called excitement of that Brazilian tour. A gift to ground me. A valuable gift to help me stay balanced.

* * *

After one of our shows in Brazil, the record company set up a big press party for us backstage. MTV, TransAmerica radio, and many music magazine writers were there. Knowing that we were interested in yoga and spirituality, the record company made the party themed, with Indian foods, music, posters of Hindu deities, and even a nationally famous yogini palm reader named Regina Shakti.

I was excited to see a palm reader, and I beelined toward her. She started telling me all about the present tour I was on, its success, and how I would travel all over South America and influence many people even outside of

Brazil. She smiled and said I would have many subsequent travels through South America—then her face puckered. She shook her head and said, "But you will get in a tragic car accident." I froze, remembering the palm reader in West Bengal. Then I grabbed her by the wrist and dragged her to Porcell. I grabbed his hand and said, "What about him? Will he get into a tragic car accident?"

She nodded. I thought, *Maybe the band will get into an accident on tour. I should have them all get their palms checked out!* As I walked her over to our drummer and second guitarist to check their palms, she shook her head. "Not these two. They will be fine. I stood perplexed. *Okay, maybe it won't be a band tragedy.*

*   *   *

I've been famous within certain circles since I was nineteen, but nothing compared to my fame in Brazil. Fans found out about our hotel and slept in our lobby to get our autographs as we checked out in the morning. Bodyguards surrounded our SUV when we got out to visit record stores in malls for autograph signings. Women threw themselves at me. Fans rocked our Mercedes Sprinter when we showed up to concerts. I signed more CDs, body parts, clothing, and tour posters than I ever had.

Many devotees of Krishna who were living in ashrams came to greet us and support us. We were also pretty popular in Germany, but things were different in Brazil. Germans were more skeptical of our spiritual message, but Brazilians loved it. Jesus, Krishna, the Buddha—Brazilians were cool with whatever. When we arrived at an airport gate, Brazilian fans greeted us with a big stand-up kirtan and offered us flower garlands and homemade prasad. It was an overwhelming lovefest.

One elder devotee sat with me in private after a press conference at the Rio Krishna temple. His name was Govinda. He was in his fifties, and his hair was gray. He spoke in English with a strong Portuguese accent and was broad-chested and strong. His face was joyous yet weather-beaten from years of tropical sun. He was soft-spoken and had deep wisdom, and we immediately engaged in deep conversation as if we were old friends. He started to elaborate on the concept of fame. I sat quietly and listened attentively because he spoke without ego or pretense.

"The sages of ancient India call fame *pratishtha*," he said. "It is one of the biggest intoxicants out there. Worse than hard addictive drugs. Yet like a hard drug, it gives a high higher than you could ever imagine. Like the addictive drugs, fame delivers such a terrible bottoming out that one needs to medicate or be miserable."

He explained that once you mix in envy of others, a fear of losing one's fame, and the media sometimes speaking ill of you, you have a cocktail of potential anxiety, distress, fury, and sadness.

According to the yogic tradition, the soul takes birth in the material world because we don't want to live in reality. We are small—infinitesimal parts of something much bigger. We are not the center. We are meant to serve the center.

"This desire to be the center is the cause of all our pain because it is, in fact, not based in reality. Do you understand, Raghunath?"

I nodded.

"If we have money, we can easily use it to convince people of our greatness," he continued. "If we are attractive, we use our body as a currency. If we are clever or charming, we use it to attract people to us and impress them. But we are not the center of the universe, so no matter how many people we fool into worshiping us, we will always feel like imposters. An imposter can never be peaceful in the world. Never, Raghunath, as imposters are always in fear that they will be found out. Deep down, we know our frailty and our pretense."

He added that wealth, beauty, knowledge, and fame were gifted to us, but they were not ours. They, like our body, were merely on loan to us.

"After all, Raghunath, how famous can you be? How long will it last? It all gets taken from us. We are forgotten in a few years. We are like fireflies compared to Krishna, who is like the sun. We are just sad imposters of the Divine Being."

I understood the illusion of fame. It had beat me up previously, before I lived in the ashram. I gave it up and the universe gave it back—bigger than it had been.

"Govinda-ji Prabhu," I said, "can you give me any advice for this tour, where fame is bigger than I've ever had?

"Use fame to serve and it will serve you," he said quickly. "If not, fame will use you. You will be a slave to it, pathetically trying to keep it. You will think you're better than others. See this fame as a gift on loan to you to do good in the world. Don't use it to manipulate others, especially women." He smiled. "God has given you two gifts, Raghunath, the highest being transcendental information, the second being popularity and influence. Use them both to serve God, not to compete with God, and your life will have genuine success."

A few days later, we played a concert at a club in Belem, the gateway to the Amazon River. The club held five thousand people, and it was sold out. We pulled up to the backstage entrance. The tropical heat was just breaking as the sun started to set. Standing on the side of the stage, I looked at all the people who were looking up at me in anticipation. They saw me as a type of demigod. Fans want to worship so badly. I remembered the talk Govinda-ji and I had had. It was the desire of the soul to give love, respect, and honor, but often we gave that love to those who were less than worthy of receiving it. We directed our love not to saints or people with spiritual integrity but to musicians, athletes, or Hollywood stars. A full surrender to false idols, people who themselves might be lost, broken, and spinning out of control. The idols took the fans' desire to love and hoarded the honor for themselves instead of realizing that fame was the honor of God, who was working through them.

I had a strong desire to hoard that honor as well. "See! Notice my greatness!" my ego shouted. "I've been telling you all along!" But my significance was not coming from their worship of me. My significance and joy came from using what I had to give back. Could I move forward with fame but not be affected by fame? Could I be big? Powerful? Charismatic? Empowered on the stage? Would I use that gift to serve God or be God? This was the only question I needed to answer.

*   *   *

Mantra was the first record we recorded with a major label, and it was exciting how they got behind us. I was sent to Europe for a week of scheduled interviews—thirty-minute interviews for magazines, radio, and television, back-to-back, all day long every day in London, Amsterdam, and Cologne, Germany. I learned the power of leveraging my time. Many of the questions were about basic information—who was in the band, our ages, and so on. Many asked me to explain yoga and Vedic philosophy and what life was like as a monk. I had to learn how to concisely explain deep Vedic teachings to people who knew nothing about them. Often, the interviewers would challenge my ideas on spirituality, animal rights, reincarnation, and material indoctrination.

Fortunately, I had already challenged myself for years at that point, so I was prepared. Still, I had to be sharp and quick with my answers, so every morning after I did my japa I'd walk the streets and go through the *Bhagavad Gita* to figure out the most compelling way to succinctly express relevant ideas that didn't sound dogmatic or perfunctory. This made me dive deeper into the meaning of the texts and their relevance. I would pose challenging questions to myself. Debate myself. All of this helped strengthen my realizations and conviction. I was convinced about spiritual hope and skeptical about material existence. Because my belief system was being challenged, I was forced to understand it with a greater depth.

Interviews usually went like this:

Q: Don't Hindus believe they are God? That's much different than our Judeo-Christian theology.

A: The theistic schools of Vedic thought say we are spirit embodied. We are pure and Godlike. We are covered and we forget our real nature and foolishly identify ourselves as a temporary reality, of sex, gender, race, etc. As Christ said, "Love God with your heart, mind, and soul." That's the essence of bhakti yoga. But who is God? That information is there in the Vedas.

Q: I've read that Hindus believe in 33 million gods.

A: There is one Supreme, but yes there are many other higher powers. The Bible also speaks of angels. Don't you think they're higher powers?

Q: I can believe in a God . . . I think. I believe in man. But with so many other beings out there its almost too much. Too fantastic. Too sci-fi.

A: Let's look at this planet first. The sages of ancient India teach that everything of this world has some life or divine spark behind it. Everything has personality and beingness. Not that God is divine and everything else is a mundane backdrop. Not that everything is dead except God and man. The teachings say that trees are spiritual beings in tree bodies. Rabbits, birds, plants—they are all spiritual beings encased in different vehicles. Some beings are very obvious, like a dog.

Suppose you have three dogs. You know that each one of them is a unique being. As we become closer to our pets we notice their proclivities, desires, and personal traits. They are not things. They are beings. We fall in love with them. We give them names, sometimes dog clothing. Just as our dogs or cats have their personal traits, plants and trees are also unique individuals. You just need to hang out with plants more.

Q: Yes I do.

A: But everything—not just dogs, every cell, bacteria—is a spiritual entity.

Q: You're not answering the question though. You said there are 33 million gods.

A: Listen, I want to first explain that I'm not saying anything that's my opinion. I don't know much. I'm not coming up with this stuff. I am teaching what the Vedic tradition says. I explain what is taught, but I don't know that it's all true. I can tell you what works for me, which teachings have changed my life. I definitely do find it to be a better road map for life than the map our present culture is choosing for us. Here is what I know. I know meditation helps my life. I know chanting helps my mind become calm and controlled. I know I should control my diet, my senses, and my sexuality. I know those are healthy things for my peace of mind and well-being. I can understand that my senses are limited, and I cannot have perfect knowledge with imperfect senses. I know being regulated in my habits is healthy. I can understand that there is a higher power than me. I know I am maintained by nature and higher powers. I can understand that I'm not a body but an animating force within the body. I can understand that the body is matter in flux. It's ever changing as I sit and observe. I can understand that my mind is a subtle body and always in flux. Always changing. I know I get either positive or negative reactions to my actions, so therefore I should be careful what I do, how I speak, and what I consume through all my senses. I can go on and on with what really makes sense to me, but there are things that I cannot understand yet. I have reasonable faith that they could be true, as all I've been taught on this journey, when applied, is incredibly helpful and beneficial for my health, well-being, and peace of mind. Thirty-three million gods? Maybe.

Q: Okay, I understand. You didn't make this up, but you do teach it. I'm sure you come across people who say, "I don't buy all this 'higher power' bull."

A: You don't believe there are higher powers? You don't believe the sun is a higher power? Go stand naked in the desert. The sun is a much higher power than you. What about the ocean? The wind? The effects of the moon? They're all higher powers. Even within a select group of people, there are higher powers. One person is more educated. One is stronger. One is more artistic. Of course there are higher powers. Why is that so hard to understand?

I find it more difficult to believe that everything is dead matter. That everything is not a being but a thing. That trees have no spirit. Animals have no spirit. The earth has no spirit. It's this type of thinking that has created an ecological apocalypse that we see in front of our eyes now. Everything is just out there for us to use at our disposal and there are no consequences. Let's see where that theory takes us.

Sometimes interviews were much more challenging:

Q: So a punk is now going to speak about God. Isn't that sort of anti-punk?

A: Why? I thought punk was "no rules"? So, if there are no rules, I'll sing about whatever I want. Right? No rules.

Q: I think when you bring God into rock or punk, you hijack something great. Rock is a rebellion against these old-fashioned standards, morals, and ethics made up by some church elders trying to control the masses. Music should break down those foolish archaic belief systems. Let us just enjoy music for the sake of music without some arrogant self-indulgent holy message.

A: I'm just putting back what were the origins of music throughout the ages. Are you saying God or spirit doesn't belong in music? That I've hijacked music by singing about spiritual subjects? Historians often argue that the very origins of music globally are to

celebrate a higher power. Music has always been intimately connected with worship, ritual, appreciation,
and giving thanks. It's been like that for millennia.
What about Bach, Beethoven, Handel? Your secular
concept of music has hijacked true music.

* * *

Before we left on tour, a TV show from England came to the Brooklyn ashram
where we were living and shot a big piece on us for a youth television show
called *Passengers*. It was a popular show for teens in the UK, and it's what
prompted the UK tour. When we got to the UK, we were often stopped on
the streets, at rest stops, or at gas stations by people who had seen it. Our
performances were extra packed on all dates in England, Scotland, and Wales.

It's said that loss, distress, poverty, and heartache can throw one off the
spiritual path. I can easily see how success or good fortune can as well. This
tour was an unprecedented time for me, where it was more common to
be recognized than not. I noticed how quickly bad qualities arose in me. I
was getting proud, arrogant, entitled, and disconnected. I started getting a
little self-righteous. I was cockier with the band and less delicate with how
I treated them. The humility goggles that I had learned in the ashram had
become cracked. I started seeing myself not as a tiny spark of something
bigger but as someone who was big and destined to get bigger. I got a
beautiful wake-up call one day in Scotland.

Porcell, now with the name Paramananda, and I were walking through
the streets of gorgeous Edinburgh by its famous castle. Some people who
had seen the *Passengers* special approached us. They were excited and
asked us to sign their shirts or shake their hands. As we went by some
tourist shops, an older man working in one looked at us firmly. He was
wearing a plaid kilt, knee socks, a tam-o'-shanter, and a leather pouch
around his belt, which acted like a purse. He had reddish-white hair and a

leathery, wrinkled face. He blurted out something to us that we struggled to understand.

"Ah you ay deevotee?"

We didn't understand his accent.

"Yaneck! Yaneck!" He pointed to his collar.

"I'm sorry sir, we don't understand what you're saying," Paramananda said.

"Ah you ay deevotee?" he said again. "Yaneck! Yaneck!" And pointed again to his collar. Then he pointed to his throat.

"Oh! My neck?" I asked. "You mean my mala? Am I a devotee of Lord Krishna? Yes!"

He recognized us from our sacred neck beads. Now with a new understanding of his thick accent, communication wasn't so bad.

"I used to know George Harrison," he said. "We were friends in the '70s in England. He'd bring me to see the Krishna Swami-ji."

Paramananda and I lit up. "You're kidding!"

"No, no, me and George were mates. He used to bring us to London to visit the swami." The man in the kilt enjoyed that we were so interested and immediately dove into storyteller mode. "The swami used to ask us questions and explain how this world is an illusion, and that we are lost, trapped in our ego trying to find God. But we were in maya. Our hearts wanted God, but we were trying to find it in the material world."

I couldn't believe we had run into him. He just kept talking.

"It was in the '70s, mate. I was into lotsa sex, lotsa drugs, lotsa drinking, and lotsa rock 'n' roll. When the swami told us we were never going to find happiness there, I heard him but didn't take him that seriously. George was different. He was much more spiritual than me. He listened to the swami. He took his words to heart. I just couldn't. I was too attached." The man's excitement calmed a little, and he started to look very grave.

"The swami would take us into his room, talk to us, give us some sweets and a flower garland, and always wrap up the conversation with the same statements. 'Life is short. Take your spiritual life very seriously. Life will race by. Don't waste this human form of life,' he would say. But I was living large. We had everything at our disposal. The circles of people I used to be with. The ladies." He paused. He sighed. "You know, I had money. I lost money. I got more money. Lost money. But look at me now, mate," he paused again. His face dramatically changed from one of relish to one of remorse. "Look at me. I'm an old man. I thought I was really special. Now a moment later I'm an old man, just like the swami said. I should have listened to the swami!"

I looked at the creases on his face, his yellowed teeth, and his faded cheap tattoos. He was probably handsome as a young man, but you couldn't tell now.

I started thinking about my fame. *Big deal*, I thought. *Big deal. This is your future, Raghunath. Get over your puny success. First, you're not that successful. Second, even if you were, you'll be an old man, in a moment.*

The man shook his head. "I should have listened to the swami," he said more to himself than to us. "I should have listened to the swami!"

He turned without saying another thing and went back into the shop.

*   *   *

An exciting year passed. We went back into the studio for three months. There appeared to be a growing buzz around the band in the United States. Many of our friends' bands were blowing up to heights we never thought possible. It seemed like every musician in the mid-1990s was thinking the same thing: Will that happen to me? After all, we were in a unique industry. You never knew if you'd be plucked from obscurity and rocket to fame or stay in the proverbial garage forever.

Some friends and fans from our teenage years now had pivotal positions at record companies and could sign bands to record deals worth hundreds of thousands of dollars. Peers of ours were getting signed to record labels that discovered the likes of the Doors, Kiss, and Led Zeppelin. It was almost unreal. The excitement and anxiety of being in limbo were unnerving. We were already at a good record label. I'd spent years prioritizing focused meditation and being detached from all results, but I was attached to the desire—with good intentions—to become massive. In retrospect I see that attachment perhaps as the lesson that came to me next.

After the Vegas show, we stopped at a friend's place, where we had a phenomenal postshow home-cooked vegan feast. It was 1 a.m. by this point, and the band planned on driving through the night, heading for Salt Lake City, the next stop on our tour.

We had a slightly different lineup than we'd had in South America, with a new drummer and guitar player. Around 2:30 a.m., our driver fell asleep at the wheel of our Ford Econoline van, which was outfitted with lofts for sleeping and a trailer for gear and merch. We tumbled 150 feet down the side of a mountain and landed in a river. I was knocked unconscious when my harmonium smashed me in the eye. I woke up to hear Porcell attempting to climb up the mountain, but he was in excruciating pain and was left sincerely chanting mantras on the cliffside. He saw my head covered with blood and thought I was dead. Our young roadie, Will, looked at me and said, "Raghu, I can't feel my legs. I can't move. Am I going to be all right?" Will hadn't been around when Regina Shakti read our palms and prophesied a terrible car accident.

The van was demolished. Everything—instruments, merchandise, luggage—was tossed about, as though the van had been destroyed in a tornado. Will lay on his back, and I perched above him, looking down as our van lay sideways on the mountainside. I could see an open copy of the *Srimad Bhagavatam*, a big sacred book from India, and Will's head was pillowed between the pages as though comforting him.

"You're resting in the sacred *Srimad Bhagavatam*, Will," I said. "I think you're going to be fine."

Three of our band members were unscathed and managed to climb up the embankment in the dead of night and flag help. Porcell and I were admitted to the hospital and treated and released. I had a severe sprain and wasn't able to walk for four months, but nothing was broken. Will broke his neck. The doctors said they'd never seen anyone recover so quickly.

So it was tragic for all, but no one died, just as both the Brazilian palmist and the West Bengal palmist had predicted.

In these tragedies, aspiring transcendentalists can find gold. I took this as a sacred sign that I needed to get more focused on my spiritual life again.

*   *   *

A year before the accident, we were on tour in the United States and wanted to stay at an ashram after a show instead of a hotel. We called ahead, but no one was awake when we arrived late at night. Instead, they left directions that explained which bunks we could stay in. As we were turning on the lights and getting settled, a holy man walked in. He gracefully floated in the door, offering namaste, and I bowed and introduced myself. He was small with a saintly face. At first I thought he was from India. "My name is Radhanath Swami. Welcome. How can I serve you?"

The swami's name and reputation preceded him, although I had never met him. He gave us sacred food and sat us down, making us feel welcome and loved. I knew he ran an ashram in India, but I had never visited it. I asked him how he got into bhakti. His story took about four and a half fascinating hours. Later it became his bestselling book *The Journey Home: Autobiography of an American Swami*.

I hadn't seen or heard from him since that auspicious meeting, but I knew he lived primarily in Mumbai at the ashram he directed. After the accident, I remembered his focus, connection, and love, and I decided to track him down. The tour was canceled, and I had some issues with my body that I wanted to take care of. But I also had some holes in my heart.

I called Mumbai, reached him, and asked whether he remembered me. I told him about our situation with the band, the accident, and how I felt my consciousness needed some realignment.

"Perhaps, Swami-ji, I could come to India and find a place to a water fast and just heal my body gently," I said. "At the same time, I feel like my soul needs regrounding. This music business is riddled with illusions, hopes, and promises of material satisfaction." There was a pause. "Hello?" I asked. "Are you still there?"

"Raghunath, of course I remember you. Can you get here by tomorrow?"

I thought for only a moment. "Yes. Yes, I can," I replied.

"Just come. Let me know your flight number. We will make all arrangements," he said, as though he was expecting my call. I hadn't been to India in almost four years, and I hadn't been a monk for three. I was in the midst of a massive spiritual download—the loudest message being that I couldn't help anybody if I couldn't help myself. All the benefits I could give through music, lyrics, and so on wouldn't make much of a difference if I couldn't apply this stuff to my own life. If I was getting swept away by big maya, what kind of example could I be?

I flew to India the next day and met the sacred swami, who on my request sent me to water fast for eleven days at a yogi's ashram somewhere in Maharashtra. For the success of the band, it was everything I shouldn't have been doing. It was a critical time. Our newest CD, *Beyond Planet Earth*, had just been released, and the marketing and publicity team was pushing it to the press. We were supposed to get out and work it. Perform. Interview. Instead, I was sitting on a rickety train, heading south to a random Indian village outside of Pune. Nothing about it made material sense, yet I desperately needed to reintegrate with my soul. The band couldn't tour anyway. Porcell was still on his back, in pain, recovering but still recuperating. It was hard for him to do anything. The car accident put the kibosh on all our plans.

It is said that when Krishna likes you, he gives you whatever you want. And when Krishna loves you, he takes it all away. That's how I felt about the car accident. It was what I needed to start refocusing on who I was and what I wanted. It helped me realize that there was always a loving director in my life, moving me, inspiring me, leading me, and watching over me. Not giving me necessarily what I wanted but always giving me what I needed.

When I returned to Mumbai after the water fast, I shadowed Radhanath Swami, who left the deepest impression in my heart. Although he had nothing, slept on the floor in a humble room, ate frugally, and rose early, he had a vision to direct transformation. He had students, hundreds if not thousands that he inspired, and they were all working eagerly on his many outreach programs—projects of spiritual transformation, ashrams, an incredible eco-village, food distribution centers, and hospitals around the world. I was blown away by how much a person could do without doing. Literally just living inspired, dreaming, and manifesting. Without trying to control. Without trying to take credit. Without trying to coerce. Lovingly moving forward and uplifting thousands. One great soul with a focused vision can do a lot.

The swami told me he wanted to show me something, and we waited by the temple gate. A car picked us up, and we drove to a hospital. He told me many of his students were doctors, and instead of working independently, they decided to join together and create a team with a shared vision: They could work not only on people's physical needs but also their emotional and spiritual needs, which were often a big part of a person's recovery when they are physically hurt or unwell.

"Is it exclusively for Hindus?" I asked Radhanath Swami, but I immediately felt foolish.

"No. We're all spirit souls. With bodies," he said. "When the bodies get sick, we take care of the body, and if they like, we care for the head, heart, and spirit as well. It's all needed in the hospital. Whatever tradition they're from, we're there for them.

I was impressed with the staff and their bedside manner. "This place makes me want to get sick just to come here and recuperate!" I said. When I walked into the cafeteria, I was blown away by the food services. Simple, healthy foods made fresh, as in an ashram.

"There's no 'food industry' frozen, brought-in-on-trays, microwaved, reheated, boiled-in-plastic-bags, vending-machines foods like in American hospitals," I observed.

"That is tragic nowadays, isn't it? Food is also medicine," said the swami, grinning.

This was the beginning of my sweet studentship with Radhanath Swami, who inspires and directs me to this day. He demonstrated the art of living with love despite a world moving against that current. It's important to have people in your life that you value for their integrity. Having leaders and elders that you can look up to is important. We tell ourselves to be our own heroes, but we miss out on valuable lessons taught by people who have walked these roads before us.

*   *   *

When I moved out of the ashram, I decided to get back into a physical practice, including Ashtanga yoga as taught by K. Pattabhi Jois, and Muay Thai kickboxing. I realized that Ashtanga was a misnomer, because it taught one type of pranayama and a set series of asanas in a one-size-fits-all manner. Little was taught about the other six limbs or any philosophy at that, and when compared to what I understood of yoga from living in ashrams, I found it pale. That being said, I *loved* the sequence of poses, which worked well with my body type, and I dedicated the next six years to seriously practicing it six days a week for almost two hours a day. Doing Ashtanga helped me show up on a regular basis for my body and mind, and it transformed my body.

I watched Ultimate Fighting Championship 1 and 2, and was convinced I wanted to study Brazilian jujitsu, but I wasn't sure how or where to learn. At the time it was an obscure martial art in the United States, and only a few cities had training facilities. Heading back to the ashram, I ran into none other than Harley Flannagan in the subway. He wore a jujitsu T-shirt. After exchanging greetings, he told me he was headed to jujitsu class and had been studying it for six months. I immediately followed him to the world-renowned Renzo Gracie Academy, where I met the master Renzo Gracie. Matt Serra, a professional mixed martial artist, was also there and had just received his purple belt with his brother Nick. I was in awe. I gave Renzo a copy of *Mantra* as a gesture of appreciation. He went into the back room and came out with an expensive Krugans kimono and handed it to me as a reciprocal gesture.

"Renzo, you don't have to do this," I said. "This kimono is expensive and this CD I get for free to give out."

"Here at this academy, it's like the church," he said. "Sometimes you give to the church, and sometimes the church gives to you. Please take it as a gift."

I was inspired, and so began my passion for jujitsu.

In 1999 I decided to get out of New York and I moved to south Santa Monica, six blocks from the beach, what the old skateboarders called Dogtown. I eventually started jujitsu with the world-famous Jean Jacques Machado, who was part of the original Gracie team that came to Southern California. After receiving my purple belt, I started leaning more into no-gi grappling, which is done without kimonos. My yoga practice, pranayama practice, a ninety-five percent raw-food diet, and lots of juice and water fasting gave me an athletic edge even though I had never been a natural athlete. The diet, fasting, and breathing techniques I practiced for health kept me lean with indefatigable stamina. Eddie Bravo, who became a well-known jujitsu instructor, was a purple belt when I was a blue belt. He was about my size and became a good model for me to follow and train with at Jean Jacques Machado's academy. His techniques were creative, unique, and out of the box. I appreciated that.

Joe Rogan was also training there and appreciated Eddie's style of fighting. When Eddie got his brown belt after putting in a long time as a purple, he went to Brazil to fight Royler Gracie, who was considered one of the best no-gi grapplers in the world. When he defeated Royler using his signature techniques, it rocked the Brazilian grappling community. When he returned to Southern California, Jean Jacques gave him a black belt immediately, and Eddie started teaching no-gi grappling at the Bomb Squad, a little Muay Thai gym in Hollywood. A handful of senior grapplers who were into no-gi fighting also went with him, including me and Joe Rogan. This was the birth of 10th Planet Jiu Jitsu, which was an entirely parallel system of no-gi grappling based on Eddie's creative genius. I had the great fortune of training with all of these cutting-edge fighters, who kept pushing this fighting style to the next level.

After years of practicing yoga, I was asked by one of my teachers if I would sub for their yoga classes when they went away on vacation. I considered myself a natural teacher and speaker, but I had never *taught* yoga. I just practiced it a lot, knew the philosophy pretty well, and could explain it.

I was honored but a little nervous. I kept my yoga practice more like a meditation. Ashtanga was done silently, or in the class I had recently been taking, they played an infinite *om* or the *Vishnu Sahashranam* in the background. How was I going to teach in a gym?

"I'll do it for you, but only if I can bring my harmonium and chant in class," I said. "That would keep me grounded and connected."

"Sure. I guess that would work." She had me teaching at five places in the Los Angeles area, and each place hired me that day. Overnight I had a new career teaching yoga. I found I loved teaching yoga more than I loved being on stage with a band. This launched a new life for me as a passionate yoga teacher, specializing in advanced asanas, philosophy, and bhakti. I slowly started to do fewer and fewer things with the band, and I became more dedicated to my teaching of yoga and furthering my martial arts. Within a short time I started taking groups of yoga students to India to holy places that I loved visiting when I was younger. I wanted them to experience the magic that I experienced as a pilgrim as opposed to a tourist.

*　　*　　*

Tirumalai Krishnamacharya was an erudite Vedic pandit, Sanskrit scholar, yoga guru, and master of logic and debate. His two disciples, B. K. S. Iyengar and K. Pattabhi Jois, spread yoga all over the world. The hybrid of their two practices was what the West called Vinyasa yoga, and this was what I taught. By 2011, I was traveling internationally to teach at workshops and festivals, everywhere from Jakarta, Berlin, Stockholm, and Singapore to Bali, Vancouver, New York City, Florence, Zurich, and of course, cities in Nepal and India—still my favorite places because of the rich culture that was there for those who looked.

I had heard that Krishnamacharya, who worshiped Krishna, had also taught secret pranayamas. I needed to find these out. One day I was visiting Radhanath Swami's ashram in Mumbai with many of my students when I heard that an elderly disciple of the late Krishnamacharya was also visiting with his wife. They were both saintly and had studied privately with Krishnamacharya for over three decades. It was said they knew hundreds of asana sequences for yoga therapy, as well as secret pranayamas, and were the most authorized teachers of his tradition. I was enthralled and excited. On top of this, he was a bhakti yogi! What were the secret pranayamas? I remembered the days when I hunted mystical breathing techniques, and now I felt like I was finally going to get answers to my prayers. I was still interested in personal mantras. Did these pranayamas give insight into the minds of others? Psychic powers? It was said that pranayama could transform us twice as much as our physical yoga practice.

I had already seen the magic that asanas can do for the body. What could these breathing techniques accomplish in terms of my potential?

The next day, Radhanath Swami formally introduced me to the great yogi and his wife, as they were guests at his temple. The yogi was thoughtful, animated, and bright-eyed. He and his wife were dressed in traditional clothing. I touched his feet and told him how honored I was to meet him and how I respected his years of dedication to the physical and mystical practices of yoga and his devotion to God. He folded his hands and gave me a head bobble of acceptance with humility. "By the mercy of guru and Bhagavan," he humbly acknowledged.

"Oh, Maharaj," I said addressing him honorifically. "I'm here in Mumbai with my students, but we'd be honored to have you teach us a class if you have time." It was a bold petition. "We would never get the honor to hear from a respected soul like you, and I'm like a bug in my yogic education compared to you. I'd be honored and thrilled if you could teach my students a yoga class." I paused. "Even part of a yoga class. Like some . . . pranayamas?" There. I had said it. "I've heard your teacher Krishnamacharya had some . . . secret pranayamas he'd share with some of his students."

"Yes, there are many pranayamas that most don't know about," he said. "I will come visit you in your class in the morning. I'd like to see your teaching."

I was humbled if not humiliated to hear that response, but maybe I could still learn something if he was in an eager mood. The next morning, he showed up with his wife and sat down on some chairs I'd left for them.

I introduced and honored him and finally spoke to him personally. "We'd be honored to have you lead the class today."

"You start, Prabhu-ji, and perhaps I will do something at the end," he said.

I nodded, attempted to encourage him again, and when he refused and insisted I continue, I looked to him for his blessings. Then I sat with the students to chant our opening mantras. We started with a mantra that called the divine energy into our life. The names in the mantra were the different names of Krishna, divine sounds describing divine attributes. It was a perfect mantra to chant to prepare the mind before starting our physical practice and our breathing.

This ancient mantra was sung by the great queen of the *Mahabharata* named Draupadi. The queen was in a dangerous and humiliating situation. She was publicly dragged into the court by the vile demand of Prince Duryodhana. He had always desired Draupadi, and to crush her spirit and make her surrender to him, he had her dragged into the royal court in front of Duryodhana's father, court ministers, the grandsire, sages, and even Draupadi's own father and five husbands. The king was blind, because of not only his childhood birth defect but also his spiritual blindness, which was due to being overly affectionate for his heinous son, who ruled the kingdom with his lower passions and was envious of his pious cousins, the Pandavas.

Duryodhana was the archetype of lust, greed, and avarice. He was a spoiled brat and was bent on conquering the heart or body of Draupadi. At this moment, she was violently dragged into the court and given the option of being either Duryodhana's slave concubine or his chief queen. In response to her loud refusal, Duryodhana decided to publicly strip her and humiliate her in front of the court. Because his father was the king, even dharmic members of the court had their hands tied and could not remonstrate their objection. Draupadi, in desperation, called out to the elders, but they too looked to the ground, toward the king, and back to the ground again. She called to the king, but he looked away, uncaring and cold, with a strong desire to please his son's whims. She called out to the great sages, but they also did not give her any comfort or protection. For diplomatic reasons, even her warrior husbands, the Pandavas, could not step in. All the people of this world having let her down, one after another, including state leaders, religious leaders, and family members, she reached her hands toward the sky in surrender. The noble queen trusted that whatever tragedy she was going through, her life was in divine hands. She knew that nobody in the world could give her shelter. From a material paradigm, it is destitution, a hopelessness in an unjust world.

But Draupadi's uplifted hands represented something much more. She was a lady of divine caliber. When the people in charge of providing and protecting dropped the ball and turned their backs on her, she entered a new spiritual dimension. There was no safety anywhere in this material world. Indeed, as she was calling out for help with one hand, she clutched her sari with the other, as the mighty strength of the prince and his brother tore at her cloth. This signified a partial surrender for the queen. Reaching out, yet desperately holding on. Finally, when her two hands lifted toward the sky, trusting that her life was in divine hands, room was left for divine magic to happen. With both hands raised, and in a state of total vulnerability, she called out a prayer, a mantra to the divine person whom the wise had always taken shelter of. She sang *Sri Krishna Govinda Hari Murari, Hey Natha Narayana, Vasudeva.* Krishna then gifted Draupadi an unlimited sari, so as she was being disrobed, she was never naked. As the cloth was being pulled from her body, it was replenished, and she spun with her hands in the air as if pulling from a massive roll of paper towels, until the perpetrators realized there was no end to this mystically long sari. With hills and mountains of sari on the ground and Draupadi still standing majestically with her hands in the air, spinning in circles, reaching to God, Light, and Truth, Lord Krishna protected her in the darkest hour.

It was by hearing these stories repeatedly that we learned that we had shelter in times of great tragedy and destitution. I could not mask my pain. I could not drink, fornicate, or shop my pain away. I had to face my pain and call divine inspiration and light into my life—to refocus my lenses and see my darkest moments as the greatest gift. And in that gift an opportunity for a resurrection of my spiritual life. My faith got stronger. I became fearless. I became free, knowing that I had only one true master and lover in this world. And that master was a sweet, loving protector of those who were destitute.

I looked over at the elderly yogi. He nodded and smiled as I chanted. Surely this mantra had been one of the most popular in India for at least five thousand years. He clapped and looked lovingly at his wife. I kept looking over to see if he would like to speak, but he gestured with his hands as if to say to continue. So, I continued. I led the class through a strong Vinyasa yoga class, leaving time at the end as I brought people to sit.

"Before savasana, Maharaj, would you like to give the class a recommendation or some instructions? Perhaps teach us some pranayamas?" My eyebrows lifted hopefully.

"Raghunath, that was just fine." He head-bobbled. "Thank you so much. I will come back tomorrow."

Hearing this, I thought there was some hope to learn some of the esoterica from this man who remained in my mind a valuable holder of the holy grail, or a combination lock to a treasure chest.

The next day, he returned with his wife. Same time. Same chairs. Same nodding and same encouragement for me to sing and start class. Same chanting. Same head nodding and sincere smiling. I sang, and the two of them looked amused and perhaps proud that some Westerners were chanting with deep love. Again, after class, I invited him to teach and speak. Yet again, I was disappointed when he said, "Everything you have done is wonderful. This is very nice."

Another day had gone by and no secret pranayama. He said he'd come again the next day. This was my last hope. Instead of waiting for class to end, I humbly petitioned him at the beginning of the class. I stood up from my harmonium when he came into the room. I spoke from the bottom of my heart. "Please, Maharaj, we are fools; please share with us. Please, for a little while only, perhaps you can teach us something from your sacred lineage that we don't know. Something your teacher in his vast wealth of knowledge has taught you. Anything you like. Or even some"—I paused and looked at him lovingly—"some secret pranayamas."

His face lit up, and he glanced at his wife and back to me. "Every day I have come here and seen you sing these mantras, these prayers, trusting that Bhagavan Sri Krishna will take care of you. I witness your students sing, and I see you sing with this love, reverence, and trust. The *Yoga Sutras* in two places mention this verse. Do you know? Ishvara pranidhana. Are you knowing?"

I nodded. "Yes, it means to give your prana, or your life air, to Ishvara, the Supreme Controller, or donate your life air or your very breath to God."

He looked at me and all the students. "Don't you understand, Raghunath? You've been doing this all along. This is the most secret of all pranayamas."

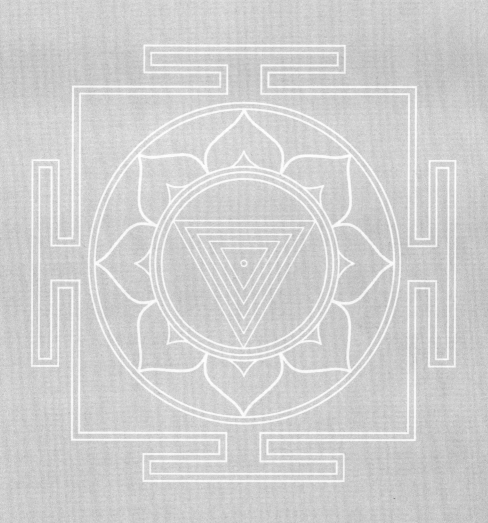

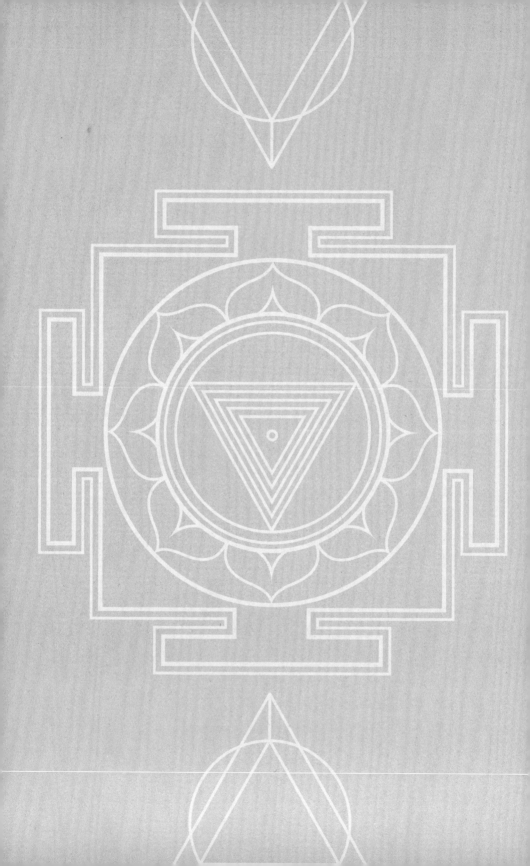

EPILOGUE

It was 2015. I had been teaching yoga since 2003. I had been taking groups of students to India since 2007, visiting holy places, temples, and people. I'd gotten married. I'd raised my wife's two little boys and had three children of my own with her.

I was leading a big group of US and European students through holy places in northern India and bringing my ten-year-old daughter for her second trip. We'd started a farm/retreat center in Upstate New York near the Berkshires to teach yoga asanas and bhakti and hold kirtans in a beautiful and natural setting. We did a lot of traveling with the kids, but India was not a tourist location for us. It was a pilgrimage. For a kid, it was an adventure to another world. We hustled to JFK Airport, taking the Amtrak to the city and finally making it on board our United flight.

Thank God I got the aisle seat, I thought, thoroughly exhausted from the trek. *I still have nine thousand miles to go before we reach Indira Gandhi International Airport.*

My daughter was excited, looking around and playing with the in-flight TV screen. We were about to begin a sixteen-hour nonstop flight to New Delhi.

"Sit and chant four rounds of the *Mahamantra* on your mala before any of those movies go on," I said sternly but with a smile. She politely obeyed. I didn't look like a sadhu anymore. And controlling my five kids was as difficult as controlling the five senses, if not more so. I had been taking the kids on my annual pilgrimages in rotation to create healthy samskaras for them. To them, the holy places were normal. Puja, bathing in sacred rivers, temple worship, dancing in kirtan, offering food with love, serving others, bowing down, singing freely in the streets with their hands in the air, being free to cry and laugh out loud—this had all become normal for them. I prayed that it would last.

I was dressed in sweats and a T-shirt to make for a comfortable flight. I had been given the karmic gift to be able to fall asleep in my seat with my legs crossed like a mystic for nine hours straight on these late-night flights. Stretching, blinking, rested, I woke up perhaps over Istanbul, Moscow, or Warsaw. Who knew? Across the aisle, a young Indian man, probably thirty years my junior, was dressed in a US collegiate hoodie and sweatpants himself. He was wide awake with his reading light on. I loved speaking to Indians to see where they were at, to see if they were still connected to the culture or had traded in that diamond for the broken glass of full-blown American consumerism. I was always amazed that many were still deeply connected, and how their training, or at least the sweet impressions in their mind from childhood and Vedic teachings, still held a directional pull in their life.

Whenever I saw Indians in the United States, be they university students, engineers, or gas station owners, I brought up the *Gita*, pilgrimage, holy places, and kirtan, and more times than not, they lit up. Then I would break out a little Hindi to have a little party, talking about sacred persons, places, and things and our favorite Indian sweets. It was always fun for everyone.

I was curious about the young man across from me. To me it seemed like he was born and raised in the United States. I wondered where his head was. He was dressed very American. He was alert at this late hour, reading some Star Wars novel. I thought I'd pick his brain.

"Excuse me, are you from India or America?" I said.

He smiled. He was good looking and could have been a Bollywood celebrity. My question seemed reasonable, as he was wearing a Penn State Nittany Lions football sweatshirt, with matching sweats, a Philadelphia Phillies baseball cap, and some type of expensive, high-tech Nike high tops that I was too old to understand or care much about.

"The US," he said softly. "I was raised in the US, but my parents are from India." He pointed over to his sleeping older parents. "They came to America in the late 1970s."

"Why did they come?" I asked, seeing that he seemed eager to engage in conversation with me.

"For a better financial future. They struggled in India and got the lottery to come," he said referring to the immigrant lottery the US offers to those who want to become citizens.

"Were they professionals?"

"No, they did anything to raise me and my older brother," he said with pride. "Literally anything. The US affords people like my parents upward mobility that wasn't available for them back home."

I nodded, as a parent appreciating what parents do for their children and the love that was behind it.

We were both leaning in to each other, happily engaged in conversation from both of our aisle seats. The flight attendant walked by and asked if we needed anything.

"Coke," he said.

"I'm good."

"And what do you do for a living? Are you at the university?" I asked, looking at his outfit.

"I've just graduated and become a dentist."

"That's incredible. But I'm going to give a lot of credit to your parents!" I said coyly, looking at him as a parent myself.

"*Please* give the credit to my parents. If it wasn't for them and their life-long sacrifice, I don't know where I would be. I'm in great debt to them. If you knew how much they struggled when they got to the States, you would have even *more* appreciation."

"And your brother?" I asked. "What about him? What is his career path?"

He paused. "He too was a dentist." His face slightly changed from a cheerful smile to a more pensive smile with pursed lips, along with a nodding head but a slightly furrowed brow.

That made *me* pause. "And why do you say *was* a dentist? Did he give up that profession for another?" I think I was hitting a raw nerve.

He smiled again, but this smile wasn't organic. He put on that smile as a teenager puts on a suit for a job interview, a suit he's not comfortable in. His mind seemed filled with thought traffic.

"Yes. He did give it up." He paused. "That's why I'm going to India now."

My daughter woke up. "I chanted my four rounds earlier, Dad! I'm gonna watch *Nacho Libre* now, okay?" she said.

"Why are you going to India now?" I asked.

"My brother has decided at this young age to take sannyasa. Do you know what that means?" he asked, thinking I was a tourist.

"Yes. I do," I said with a sober face. "He's giving up the world. He's giving up his material life with formal vows."

"Yes, it means he's giving up the material world. In our particular tradition, when that God calling comes and we answer it, we break all ties with our loved ones." He paused again.

"Not every tradition is like that in India," I said. "I have been practicing bhakti yoga for thirty years, and my teacher is currently visiting his father now. My teacher will come, share some intimacy or some wisdom teachings with his father, and then go back out to wander and teach. The meaning of sannyasa in the *Gita* is that you give up the desire for sense gratification within the heart. So, it's not necessarily where you are, or whom you're associating with, but keeping our consciousness focused on 'I'm not here to take from this world; I'm here to give back.'"

Then I quoted verse 6.1 from the *Bhagavad Gita* in English: "One who is unattached to the fruits of his work and who works as he is obligated is in the renounced order of life, he is the true mystic, not he who lights no fire and performs no duty."

"That's the deepest meaning of sannyasa according to the *Gita*," I said.

Afterward, I felt stupid. He was going through an emotional moment and experiencing great loss, and I just wanted to rub it in his face that I knew something that he didn't—and perhaps to prove my depth of understanding of India's literature and traditions. I was foolish, and I missed the point. This guy was revealing his heart to me, and I wasn't even present enough to empathize with him.

I started again a little humbled. "I'm sorry, I understand that there are many traditions in India. I didn't mean—"

"My tradition is different," he said. "When one takes sannyasa, the familial connections are totally over. We are all going to India to lovingly say goodbye to him."

As a father, I paused. I furrowed my brow and nodded but needed more information.

"Were you and your brother close?"

"Intimately," he said. His face was serious.

"Are you hurt or . . . angry that he's leaving?"

He ingested and inhaled my question. "At first I was," he said, exhaling. "I was very angry. I felt abandoned. Worthless. I blamed myself. But this was all self-indulgent whining. In our culture"—he spoke firmly here, as if preaching—"we understand that the spiritual calling is the highest of all callings, and that everything and every person in this world is temporary

339

and secondary to our original relationship with Narayana, or God. When we get that calling loud enough, we must answer it." He paused again. "My brother was a dentist, but he was always absorbed in spiritual matters, even as a child. He went through the motions in junior high school and high school. His grades were impeccable. He was athletic. He's handsome. But he knew . . . we knew he had a higher calling." He paused again. "It was only our selfishness that upset us. It was our loss. It hurt us all when he made that decision to leave. So, we dug deep and realized this is the most noble choice he could make, even though he didn't fulfill our desires of what we wanted from him. We knew this would fulfill his deepest desires. And this is the beauty of our path. We will give up what's good for what is great. He is not giving up much. Material life, I'm sure you know, is like having pocket change. With all its glamour, it is riddled with complications, heartbreak, drudgery, and exhaustion . . . for what? He is giving up pocket change for a massive inheritance of spiritual wealth and joy. You lived in some ashram, hmm?"

He lifted his head and raised his eyebrows, waiting for an acknowledgment. I nodded.

"Then you know the joy of a regulated life, meditation, rising early, and inner work. His life will not be static and dreary. It will be ecstatic and inspired. This I know." He was firm in his conviction of this, and I could see his pride, if not his envy, for his brother's choice. "This is why we're doing this trip today."

He looked over to his sleeping parents. His father wore a Nehru-collar kurta with white pajama pants, and his mother wore a Punjabi outfit. Their skin was old, like well-worn leather, and they were beautiful like sleeping children.

"My parents and I want to support his choice, so we are going to say goodbye."

He was speaking like a wise man, but I could tell his heart still hurt.

"And now what will you do?" I asked.

"We will go and say goodbye and tell him how proud we are. I will do something different on my return. I will move back in with my parents, continue my dentistry, but take care of them now that they are older. My father suffers some ill health and cannot work." He took a big inhale. "This is something I find heartbreaking about your culture"—he looked more deeply at me—"the parents give you everything when you are a vulnerable child, and you give nothing back to them when they are old and vulnerable."

He was schooling me. I was fifty-plus, an international speaker, a sought-after yoga teacher people searched out for the inner meanings of Vedic wisdom, and I was about to get schooled by a twenty-two-year-old newly graduated dentist. I took a deep breath and listened—and made a mental note to check in with my mom as soon as the plane landed in New Delhi.

"I'm going to care for them until they die. These are our parents!" He raised his voice. "They are not disposable. We take them, use them, and toss them out when they can no longer give. As a young man in America, I find it disheartening that people are so spiritually disconnected."

"That's beautiful," I said. "I hope my children feel the same way. I'm sure your parents are proud . . . of both of you. If you don't mind me saying, *I'm* proud of both of you."

I looked happily over at my daughter, who'd fallen back asleep.

"Hey bro, what is your name?" he asked

"Raghunath," I said.

He smiled, as Raghunath is a beloved name in Hindu culture. "You know that's a name for Lord Rama, right?"

"Yes, yes." I head-bobbled and smiled. "Raghunath *Das* actually.

He appreciated my head bobble and my joking Indian accent.

"So, it's not Raghunath—it's the servant, or the das, of Raghunath."

"That's right. My name means the servant of Raghunath, or the servant of God."

341

"This is the problem nowadays in culture, and it's ruining our planet," he said casually and confidently. "People don't want to serve God. They want to *be* God." He paused, rearranged his sitting posture, and looked more deeply at me. "Wouldn't you agree?"

"Yes. Desperately trying to be the center and not serve the center."

The plane landed roughly, giving our bodies a shake, and a few of the passengers clapped. The Indira Gandhi Airport was like a glamourous mall compared to New Delhi's uninspired and stodgy airport in 1988.

Over were the days of the one-lane, potholed road to Vrindavan. There was a beltway around New Delhi, and the Yamuna Expressway—complete with Starbucks at the rest stop—drastically cut our drive time. As we cruised down the massive five-lane highway at a hundred kilometers an hour, I held my daughter's hand. She was excited for the pilgrimage, and she was about to meet thirty-four of my American yoga students. Despite the infrastructure upgrades, the smell of burning dung still lingered in the air.

Taking my kids to India each year has been the greatest satisfaction I could ever have. Having them create a new normal and be acquainted with sacred people and sacred villages has been the most satisfying parenting experience. How can I ever pay back all the people, teachers, and caregivers who have touched my heart with this spiritual magic? I cannot pay them back. I can only pay it forward.

"First stop, Rishikesh," I told my daughter. "We're going to the Ganges."

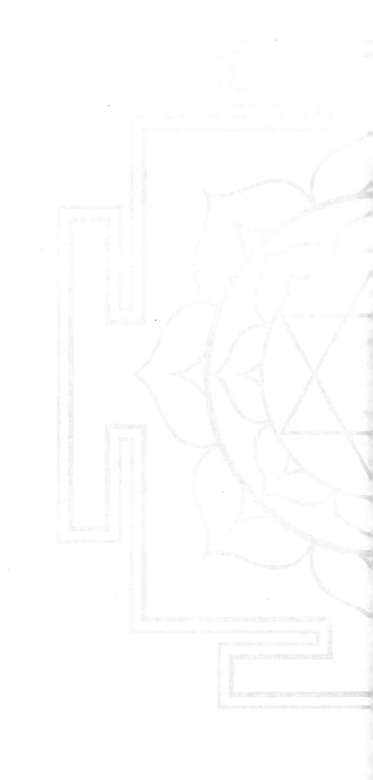

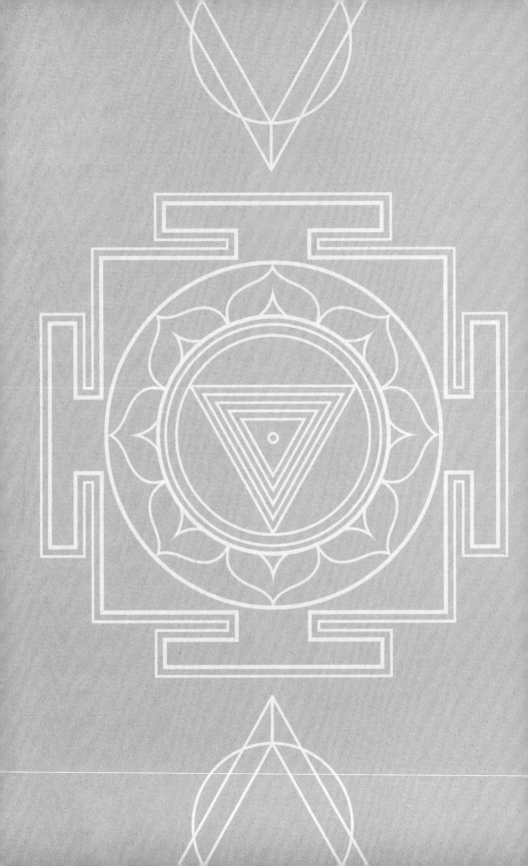

ACKNOWLEDGMENTS

Aside from all of the excellent teachers, guides, and inspirational song-writers I have met and mentioned in this book, I'd also like to thank HH Sacinandana Swami, who has helped me at the forks in my path and prayed for my good fortune. Thank you, Maharaj. I feel so fortunate to have you in my life.

Thank you to Grandma Terri, my inspirational mother and matriarch of our family. She raised seven kids, was a devoted wife, a grandmother many times over, and a great-grandmother. She has taught me so much by her example. I can't express my gratitude enough, Mom. Also, thanks to the fantastic Cappo family. I've got great siblings.

Thank you to Kaustubha Das, my bosom friend, confidant, and sounding board, who cofounded *Wisdom of the Sages* with me, and to Mara Simons-Jones, for selflessly assisting us along the way. You have been such jewels in my life. This daily offering has kept me focused through sweet and tragic times, keeping the main thing the main thing. Thank you both.

Thanks to the Mandala team, especially Raoul Goff and Phillip Jones, for believing in me and this book. So grateful for all of your feedback and encouragement.

Thank you to Tukarama Das for your deep friendship and fantastic advice, and for helping me resurrect my spiritual life in my darkest hours. I've learned so much from you and will always remain in debt for all the love and time you've given me.

Thanks to Porcell, aka Paramananda Das, for friendship, touring the world, writing, performing, and recording music with me, and living our dreams. I'm honored to have walked this path with you since our teens.

To Sammy, Walter, Mike Judge, Richie, Drew, Craig, and Tommy, who are inspired musicians and toured the world with me in Youth of Today, thank you for your friendship, creativity, and tolerance of my shortcomings. Thank you for spreading a message of light and clean living in so many dark places.

Thanks to Shelter members Ekendra Das, Krishna Chaitanya Das, Graham Land, Roy Mayorga, Adam Blake, Franklin Rhi, and the multitude of changing bandmates. You planted the seeds of bhakti and self-transformation all over the planet. I'm forever indebted to all of you.

Thank you to Saci Suta Das (aka Steve Reddy) and Keli Lalita (Kate Reddy) for what you've created, how you live, and your generosity to so many. I am so honored to be walking this path with you since Janmashtami 1988.

To Brij, my friend and the mother of my children, thank you for all of your love for, encouragement of, and belief in me.

To my children and adopted children, I love you all more than you could imagine—Sachi, Rocco, Tarun Govinda, Kishor, Damodar, Alex Claesson, and Tommy Faucett.

Thanks to Janeshwar Das for your assistance and friendship on so many of our spiritual adventures throughout India, Nepal, and Europe, which changed not only my life but the lives of so many. These pilgrimages have been some of my fondest memories.

Thank you to Mukesh and Chanchal for all of your assistance, support, and friendship traveling through India. Your deep devotion and humility is inspirational.

Thank you to Madan Mohan Oppenheimer for lasting friendship and always keeping me questioning deeper.

Thanks to Henry Schoellkopf, one of my closest friends and confidants, who's always been there for me with support and good instruction. What a wild ride this has been! Thank you for loving me and my children.

Thanks to Mukunda Kishor and family for sincerity, example, and support.

Thanks to Kent Putnam for all that you do for others.

Thanks to the late Aindra Das for instructions and inspiration.

Thanks to Shyamasundar Das, author of *Chasing Rhinos with the Swami*. The way you have lived bhakti inside and outside the box has been my inspiration.

Thanks to Ray Lego for digging up some of these great photos.

Thanks to Moby for the music, message, and example.

To my brij basi friends—Banu Nandini, Krishna Murari Goswami, Leela Vilasini, and Mohan (Radha Kunda).

Thanks to Joe Rogan and Rich Roll for support and amplifying the transcendental message of the *Srimad Bhagavatam*.

Thanks to Bob Healey for all of your input, support, and friendship.

And, in no specific order, thank you to all the special people who have touched, moved, supported, and inspired me: Indradyumna Swami; Varsana Swami; Braja Bihari Das; Radha Kunda (Chowpatty, Mumbai); Fabio (Turin, Italy); Vivi (Zurich); Amarananda Das; Chaturatma Das; Jason Golub; Vedasara Das (Atlanta); Cindy Lunsford; Bobbie Marchand; Dayal Gauranga; the late Gopal Chandra Prabhu; Alexandra Moga; the Mayapuris and all of their families; Gaura Vani, Vrinda Buchwald, and family; Madhava Das; Radhikesh Das; Lori and Brian Pagliaroni; Drew Lawrence; Sri Govinda and Shyamsundari of Shyam Ashram (Cali, Colombia); Mallory McGavin; Jayashri Triolo; Kelly Skinner; Jiva and the Bhakti Recovery Group; Jahnavi Harrison; Tarak (Italy); Tara Das (Mayapur); Narayani Seifert; Katie Ribsam of Yoga Bohemia; Andrea K. from Sangha Center for Yoga and Wellness; Zeb Homison from Yoga Factory (Pittsburgh); Tim from Boston Yoga Union; Harley Flanagan and Cro-Mags; Chris Daily; Roger and Vinnie from Agnostic Front; Kevin and 7 Seconds for the message; Louie from Antidote; Pro Bose; Revelation Records; Equal Vision Records; Keli Krishna of Podcast Farm; Jai Giridhari and Shyama; Vira and Dhyana; Rich Hornberger; Bryan Christner; Sridhar from Bhakti Fest; Perry and Lisa Julien; Sherry Sutton Photography; Jean Jacques Machado; Yogeshwara and Namamrita; Banki Bhakta Justin; Dustin (for tattoos) and Meg from Jai Yoga; Scott Bakoss of Eastern Pass Tattoo; Boofish; Jay Shetty; Ava Taylor from YAMA; Kumi from Veda Yoga Center (Culver City); Bhagavatananda (UK); the late Bri Hurley; Shrinivas from the Waitsfield Inn (Vermont); Hari Priya from Govardhan EcoVillage; Damodar and Radha from Bhava Wellness; Patrick of the Hudson Yoga Project; and Jeff and Heidi Simms.

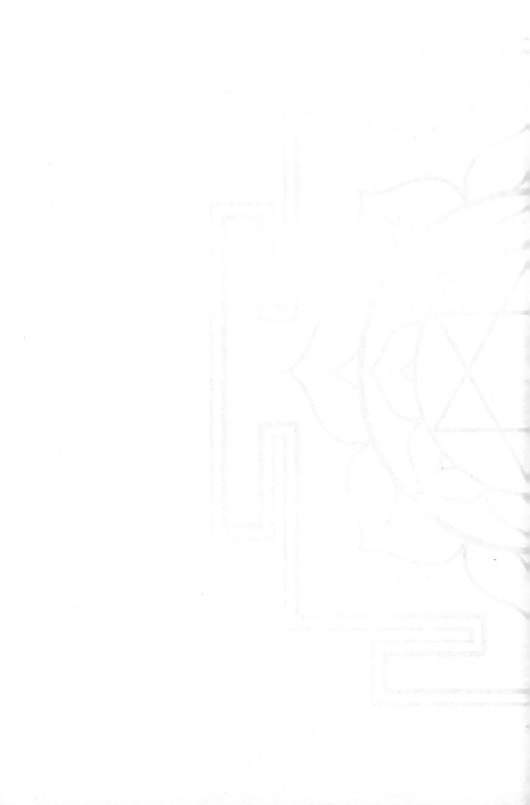

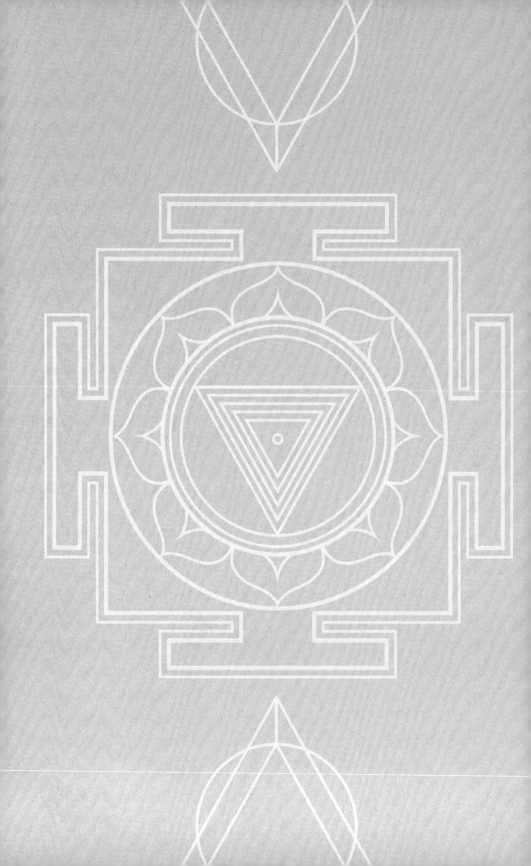

ABOUT THE AUTHOR

As a teen in the '80s, Ray Raghunath Cappo founded the hardcore punk band Youth of Today, which championed the principles of clean living, vegetarianism, and self-control. After experiencing a spiritual awakening in India, he formed a new band, Shelter, devoted to spreading a message of hope through spiritual connection. Ray currently leads yoga retreats, trainings, and kirtans at his Supersoul Farm retreat center in Upstate New York, as well as annual pilgrimages to India. He is the cofounder and cohost of *Wisdom of the Sages*, a daily yoga podcast that has been ranked No. 1 on Apple for podcasts about spirituality.

MANDALA

An imprint of MandalaEarth
PO Box 3088
San Rafael, CA 94912
www.MandalaEarth.com

Find us on Facebook: www.facebook.com/MandalaEarth
Follow us on Twitter: @MandalaEarth

Publisher Raoul Goff
Associate Publisher Phillip Jones
Publishing Director Katie Killebrew
Senior Editor John Foster
Editor Peter Adrian Behravesh
Editorial Assistant Amanda Nelson
VP, Creative Director Chrissy Kwasnik
Art Director Ashley Quackenbush
Senior Designer Stephanie Odeh
VP Manufacturing Alix Nicholaeff
Senior Production Manager Joshua Smith
Senior Production Manager, Subsidiary Rights Lina s Palma-Temena

Mandala Publishing would also like to thank Tania Casselle, Jessica Easto, Nagaraja Dasa, and
Bob Cooper for their work on this book.

Text © 2024 Ray Cappo
Foreword © 2024 Moby
Photograph on front cover © Bri Hurley
Photograph on back cover © Ray Lego

All quotes from the *Bhagavad Gita* come from the Bhaktivedanta Book Trust edition, *Bhagavad Gita
As It Is*, by A. C. Bhaktivedanta Swami Prabhupada.

ISBN: 978-1-64722-868-2

Manufactured in China by Insight Editions
10 9 8 7 6 5 4 3 2 1

Insight Editions, in association with Roots of Peace, will plant two trees for each tree used in the manufacturing
of this book. Roots of Peace is an internationally renowned humanitarian organization dedicated to eradicating
land mines worldwide and converting war-torn lands into productive farms and wildlife habitats. Roots of Peace
will plant two million fruit and nut trees in Afghanistan and provide farmers there with the skills and support
necessary for sustainable land use.